FAREWELL
Club Perma-Chub

A Sugar Addict's
Guide to Easy
Weight Loss

Jill Escher

Illustrations by Melanie Hosoda

Foreword by Jimmy Moore

DEDICATION

This book is dedicated to every frustrated dieter who has ever thought of sugar as mere "empty calories."

Designed by
A Book in the Hand
San Francisco, California

Published by Claradon Press
For more information, please contact

CLARADON PRESS
1590 Calaveras Avenue
San Jose, CA 95126
408-314-1655

• Table of Contents •

♦ Foreword ♦

The first reaction most people have when they hear the word "addiction" is hardcore illegal drugs, alcohol and other obvious bad stuff that they'd never ever engage in. But when you start talking about having an addiction to sugar, white flour, starchy carbohydrates and other foods that are wreaking havoc on the weight and health of a vast majority of the population, people immediately become defensive, skeptical and argumentative because they don't like the idea of being an addict.

You certainly can't blame them for reacting this way since all we've ever heard from our government health leaders at the United States Department of Agriculture and the so-called health "experts" over the years is that the body needs carbohydrates for fuel and you need to avoid consuming fat, especially "artery-clogging" saturated fat, if you want to be truly healthy. But what if that well-meaning advice was just plain dead wrong, and the very diet that has been promoted as "healthy" for most of your life is in fact what is keeping you fat, sick and addicted? That's precisely what Jill Escher shares in this extraordinary book you are about to read.

Take it from me, I've been there. In January 2004, I weighed in at 410 pounds, wore 5XL shirts and size 62-inch-waist pants, was on three prescription medications for high cholesterol, high blood pressure and breathing problems, and was a severely addicted carbohydrate/sugar addict at the age of 32. The only problem was I didn't know it at the time.

It was at that point in my life that I felt so incredibly frustrated by the failure of being on low-fat diet after low-fat diet with all the hunger and misery that comes with it that I decided to embark on something revolutionary that changed my life forever. I went on a high-fat, moderate protein, low-carb lifestyle change that helped me shed 180 pounds off my body, helped me come off all of my prescription medications and gave me a newfound passion for telling others about how they too can overcome their addiction and get healthy.

As Jill shares within the pages of this book, I am the host of a popular iTunes podcast called "The Livin' La Vida Low-Carb Show" (www.thelivinlowcarbshow.com/shownotes) where I have had the privilege of interviewing hundreds of the world's foremost experts on diet, health and the carbohydrate connection to obesity and chronic disease. I only wish I could have had a book like *Farewell, Club Perma-Chub* when I was going through my transformation. It would have made the journey a lot easier to endure knowing what was happening to me.

But for those of you who are currently on or considering starting your own road to better health, Jill helps you get there by dealing with the core of the addiction — sugar, white flour, processed carbohydrates, fast food and junk food — first and foremost. Because we're learning that weight loss actually begins in the mind and then manifests itself in the actions we take and how we physically change our lives.

Part of that mind renewal is realizing you have an addiction, accepting the reality of that and then beginning the difficult, yet attainable road to recovery. I've been there, Jill's been there and so have hundreds of thousands more. This book will inspire you anew to get serious about the addiction that plagues you and millions more who desperately need the central message of this book to become the theme song of their lives. Once you learn how those sugary, carbohydrate-laden foods are impacting how you think in the same manner that a crack cocaine addict responds to his drug of choice, you'll make the fateful decision to beat this addiction once and for all.

I was worth it, Jill was worth it and now YOU are worth it, too. You just need the courage of your convictions to know what is right for you — and then DO IT! Because once you start livin' la vida low-carb, ain't nothing gonna stop you from becoming the person you were always meant to be. Now get out there and GO FOR IT!

Hope you like it!

— *Jimmy Moore*

Livin' La Vida Low-Carb Blog & Podcast
www.livinlavidalowcarb.com/blog
livinlowcarbman@charter.net

• Introduction •

"The worm in the onion knows nothing sweeter."
— Yiddish proverb

I'm ready to take a life-changing journey with you, but I need to be honest and let you know that I'm hardly Ms. Original. Most of the roads we'll travel during our little adventure have already been mapped in various ways by esteemed researchers, physicians, food historians, journalists, addiction counselors and nutrition experts.

So people ask, how is my story different? Why bother writing yet another book about weight loss?

Well, first, there was the urging of several friends who wanted to know more about my weight loss "secrets." And second, because everyone else deserves to know them, too. America remains firmly gripped by epidemics of obesity, heart disease, type 2 diabetes, metabolic syndrome, cancer, hypertension and other conditions largely related to the food we eat. About 75 percent of our soaring health care expenditures are spent on these and other fairly preventable diseases. Experts have bemoaned the seemingly intractable nature of the epidemics, decrying the "lifestyles," "lack of willpower" and "poor food choices" of our pudgy nation.

But a correction is in order. I don't think we have an epidemic of poor lifestyle choices, but rather an epidemic of entirely innocent and well-meaning people not getting all the facts they should know about how some modern foods are distorting their bodies' various biochemical systems, leading to undesired and wholly undeserved weight gain.

So, I'm writing this book to shed more light on the underlying biochemical syndrome that has steadily been thickening our waistlines, but which few of us understand or know we have. Let's keep the books, websites, blogs, videos and podcasts coming until we understand the real root of our problems and the powerful shortcut to weight loss and improved health.

Though I have conducted dozens of interviews and consulted many sources (fellow research junkies can check the Resources section of the book for some of my favorites), my purpose is not to elaborately recite data and studies, but to synthesize the various strands of narrative into a tidy and accessible package most people can easily understand. My own personal story is included in the mix because I lived it and it worked. Once I figured out the real cause of my weight gain and other health problems, I cracked the weight puzzle with more ease than I thought possible.

I want the same success for you and am providing the tools you need to make it happen. When you move from the onion of deprivation diets to the apple of the new weight loss paradigm, life can become much sweeter indeed. Thanks for joining me in this adventure into freeing yourself from the most pervasive and under-recognized addiction in the world. Your life will never be the same.

— *Jill Escher*

1

Stuck in Club Perma-Chub

◆ ◆ ◆

Not long ago, I weighed 156 pounds, at least 30 pounds north of what a five-foot-tall woman of 45 years ought to. In fact, according to the standard height/weight charts used by doctors, I was considered mildly obese. I hid it well and did not look very fat, but had several Michelin Man-like rolls of chub around my middle. My upper arms were beginning to take on the shape of hanging prosciutto hams and my face was framed by a nascent double chin.

I had tried many times to lose my weight without success, so I figured I was destined, though not quite sure why, to be forever chunky. I assumed that I, whose earliest memory is that of being a two-year-old desperately prying open a small toy bottle of sugar pills in a pretend doctor's kit, was constitutionally incapable of eating normally or losing my sweet tooth. And hey, I was just too darn busy to deal with it anyway.

• The Talking Tootsie Roll •

Then one day in September 2010, I attended a large autism conference hosted by my son's school and ran into an old friend. Barbara used to be as round as a bass drum, with a cute but puffy face. Where did that person go? She had transformed from a spacious size 20 to a svelte size 6 and now was as slender as a forest nymph, with luminescent skin. I almost didn't recognize her. What on earth had happened?

"Oh, I lost 70 pounds," she said nonchalantly, shrugging her now well-defined shoulders.

"You did what? Seventy pounds!"

"Yeah, it was easy, no big deal," she shrugged again.

Easy? No big deal? How could losing all that weight possibly be easy? I couldn't even manage to shed an inch. "That's amazing!" I said. "How did you do it?"

She explained she had joined a group called Overeaters Anonymous and finally put an end to her compulsive overeating. She no longer ate sugar or white flour, limited herself to three meals a day and ate no snacks. "I've lost my cravings for them, I'm not even tempted any more," she said, gesturing toward some mini Tootsie Rolls lying on a display table behind us.

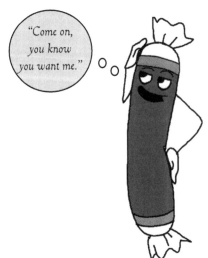

"Come on, you know you want me."

The candies did not speak to her, but to me, an inner voice buzzed, "Mmm, chocolate," as if I had no say in the matter and then, "C'mon, reach for it. Why not have just one? Just because Barbara doesn't eat them doesn't mean you can't."

"That's wonderful. I need to lose weight, too," I said as I reflexively grabbed and unwrapped the little brown corn-syrupy blob. "I eat a lot of sugar, but you know, I'm not really a compulsive overeater."

"Oh yes, you probably are," Barbara replied flatly. "You just haven't realized it yet."

I chewed my little sugar fix and thought, huh? A compulsive overeater? I didn't binge and loved nothing more than lentils with yogurt or salad for lunch. The thought of consuming plates of burritos, bags of cookies and buckets of fried chicken made me ill. No, no, not me. But nevertheless, I had to admit to this persistent subsurface urge, this craving to eat something sweet, preferably chocolatey, each and every day and often a few times a day.

In fact, I couldn't remember the last 24-hour period that had passed without munching some sort of sweet. Sometimes it was a coffee shop cookie, a mocha-flavored yogurt cup (hey, it said "low-fat"), some trail mix (M&M's must be okay if mixed with raisins and nuts) or a few squares (for starters) of a fancy European candy bar my husband left in the pantry. The variety was endless and the world offered a vast smorgasbord.

Maybe, like Barbara, I wasn't destined to live in Club Perma-Chub after all. Maybe I had a little, uh, problem that needed to be addressed.

◆ The 300-Pound Stripper ◆

Intrigued by Barbara's story, but still helplessly submitting to a daily yearning for sugary snacks, my curiosity nipped at me until I decided to log on the Overeaters Anonymous website to see if I could sample a local meeting. The next one was held the following Tuesday evening, October 5, at a small, borrowed room in a church down the road. The speaker that night was a strange-looking fellow; a gigantic, grinning man enveloped in a tent-like black suit with a black fedora atop his balding head. His girth (an airplane hangar came to mind) made his metal folding chair look tiny, like a child's.

He stood up, began speaking, and then started taking off his clothes. Huh? Nervous smiles and side glances filled the room. This was not quite what we expected. He slowly unbuttoned his jacket and then his shirt. But where was all the flesh? Instead of bulging globs of fat, he grabbed at a pillow tucked inside his clothes and placed it on his chair.

As he continued speaking, he slowly unbuckled his belt, which when unfurled was as long as he was tall. Then he pulled out another pillow and his pants fell to the floor in a puddle and then slid over his shoes. The fedora, which I now noticed was far too big for his head, came off last. Having shed the cocoon of what turned out to be his former "fat" clothes, there emerged a handsome and lean 62-year-old man wearing khaki pants and a button-down shirt tucked in neatly at his trim, belted waist.

He floated a little tap dance and laid down on the floor to do a push-up, appearing free and light. Having lost 150 pounds, he was down to about 155 and still seemed a little shocked that he now wore a medium size with no more use for the Big and Tall store. "I'm not half the man I used to be," he joked.

With the support of his OA fellowship, he had maintained his abstinence from sugar and white flour one day at a time. He stuck to his weighed-and-measured portions until the pounds melted away, revealing this fit, energetic body and a spirit gripped by a renewed zest for life. It was not his body that did the work but rather, "this stuff here, between my ears," he told our small assembly. He had not dieted — not a bit. Instead, he had found recovery from the disease that had caused him to eat compulsively.

Though our stories differed dramatically on the surface, I began to sense that just like the Stripper, some part of my eating had grown out of my control, and I too needed some sort of recovery from the disease behind my sugar-seeking behavior and not a superficial diet that simply cut calories. I began to understand that I grew heavy not because I was a weak-willed person with sloppy habits, but because I lived in a silent servitude to a need for a regular fix, just like a drug addict enslaved by cravings.

I now look back mystified to have gone so many decades oblivious to my plain-as-day sugar addiction, but I suppose I had an excuse. I had never heard of this disease, thought I actually liked sugar and naively considered refined sugar a type of food. Worse, I assumed those daily cravings were normal, but that some people — who were clearly superior to weak-willed me — possessed more willpower to resist them. And unlike drug addiction or alcoholism, chronic sugar consumption remains socially acceptable and heavily reinforced in our popular culture. That night though, I began to turn a corner. I wasn't exactly sure where I was going, but I knew it had to start with attacking my obvious chemical dependency.

• Making the U-Turn •

First, let me say a little more about my symptoms before I started my recovery program. Weight was one of my problems, but hardly the one that concerned me the most. My cholesterol was high and my doctor on several occasions urged me to take a statin drug. I demurred. She had concerns about my blood glucose level and called my pancreas (the organ that secretes the insulin hormone, which enables the body's cells to absorb glucose), "tired." I had trouble sleeping and waking up, and food cravings struck before I even stepped out of bed.

Like a crotchety old man, something always felt wrong: allergies, joint pain, fatigue. My skin was getting blotchy and I had dark circles under my eyes. My feet felt tingly in the morning and my gums were beginning to recede. My mood was generally down, but perhaps the worst symptom of all was the constant roller coaster between buzz and slump that fueled my ongoing need for the pick-me-ups provided by sweets.

I was also the classic sugar sneak. I would pat myself on the back while loading my grocery cart with fruits and veggies at the market, but then on my way to the register, feel unable to resist the impulse to pick up a box of cookies, chocolate chip "protein" bars or the like. And I was not above foraging for sweets at other people's homes, with or without their knowledge.

To make the U-turn into recovery, I needed a plan. The day after the meeting, not knowing quite what to do, I simply plucked one off the Internet. It was an outdated OA low-carb food plan called the "Grey Sheet." Though it may no longer be OA doctrine, I liked its simplicity and the way it omitted all sugar and starch, which I knew in my case fed my cravings. Four ounces of protein were allowed for breakfast, lunch and dinner, as well as one fruit for breakfast and a vegetable and salad for both lunch and dinner.

• Managing the Pains of Withdrawal •

Not surprisingly, I found the plan rather strict and ended up with slightly larger portions and a few snacks like almonds and grapes here and there, but I mainly stayed within its parameters. I bought a small kitchen scale and for about a week or two, I weighed and measured my food. That helped me grasp how much I was was really eating and helped me draw clear boundaries around the portions my body actually needed for nourishment and energy, as opposed to the inflated portions I used to inhale in response to my carb cravings.

That first week without sugar, I experienced a version of the fatigue, irritability, cravings and distraction that seemed straight out of an addiction textbook. I remember, for example, feeling at times like a snail on Dramamine, unable to rouse myself out of bed. Or just feeling numb and joyless, like my emotional inner life had flatlined. And then there were the cravings. For those dieters who pooh-pooh the idea of sugar or starch addiction, try going cold turkey and see what happens. Is that as easy as, um, pie, or are you steering your car to the nearest convenience store to find temporary relief in the shimmering cream of a Hostess Cupcake?

I latched onto some tools that helped me through. Needing moral support and steady doses of I-can-do-this-really-I-can inspiration, I dropped in on other OA meetings, read the literature, listened to a series of inspiring OA podcasts and even read parts of the famous Alcoholics Anonymous "Big Book." Each story of recovery I heard or read boosted my own confidence. And every person I met taught me something new about believing in my disease in the face of a skeptical world and about maintaining what at that time felt like a shaky sobriety.

I also found my own version of "methadone" in lots of those diet iced teas and lemonades made with little packets of drink powders. I am not proud of dousing my cravings with artificial sweeteners, but in those early weeks I must admit they helped nurse me through some rough patches.

I also needed the great savior of distraction, which I found in my work, my endless to-do list and of course, my kids. Whenever possible, it was best to steer clear of the kitchen, which remained stocked full of my husband's and kids' cookies, ice cream, bread and other high-carb treats.

Talking about my addiction and withdrawal also helped, and I was fortunate to have many patient friends willing to hear me blab endlessly about my newfound quest. The therapeutic gabbing eventually planted the seed for what became my mini-crusade to help others understand and recover from their own food-related addictions.

Each day of abstinence became easier than the last. I stuck pretty close to my food plan, preparing satisfying meals like big, chopped salads with veggies and chicken, or baked squash with salmon and spinach. I soon started losing my taste for the white stuff. Addiction had been like a ravenous little gremlin camped out in my head, barking orders about what to eat, puppeteering my hands and making me weak with cravings. Now I felt the toothy fella was finally shriveling up.

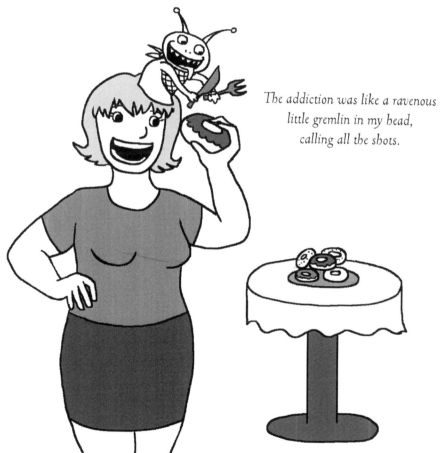

The addiction was like a ravenous little gremlin in my head, calling all the shots.

• The Sweet Taste of Victory •

They say it takes about three weeks for a habit to settle in and my case was no exception. I knew for certain my body had survived withdrawal just before the sugar addict's most dreaded holiday, Halloween. I hosted a work meeting at my house and someone on the team presented an elaborate tray of Martha Stewart-worthy cupcakes decorated with chocolate frosting and Oreo "tombstones."

Everyone "oohed" and "aahed," and normally those cute little confections would have screamed in my ear, "Must! Eat! Adorable! Cupcake! Now!" But this time, they may as well have been plump brown erasers. I took a pass and did not feel the least bit deprived. What a contrast to every Halloween in memory: instead of pilfering my kids' mini Snickers bars, I became the crazy lady handing out pencils and lecturing traumatized little ninjas and princesses about the dangers of sugar and candy.

By the time Thanksgiving came around, I happily indulged in the salads, vegetables and turkey without yearning for the stuffing, breads and pies. I was steadily losing weight at a rate of at least two pounds a week and some of my clothes were starting to hang on me like sacks. My energy was strong and steady and gone were the roller coaster highs and lows that had plagued me for years. My brain fog was lifting.

By December 7, only two months after my fateful visit to the 300-Pound Stripper, I had shed 20 pounds and was thrilled to see the number 136 show up on the bathroom scale. Aside from walking my son to school several times a week — about three slow-paced miles round trip — I hadn't exercised a bit. So much for the theory of "no pain, no gain."

Though I wasn't a regular at the gym, I did become a regular at the local produce stands, buying three or four overflowing bags of produce at a time, usually for half of what it cost at supermarkets, and I invested in the best eggs, fish, chicken and beef I could find. I delighted in the natural sweetness of food and craved dishes like salad with pear, almonds, tomatoes and chicken. Knowing my body was my own best test tube, I experimented with various approaches to foods and figured out what worked best for me.

Got Addiction?

This isn't just my story. After interviewing dozens of people with chronic weight problems, certain patterns became surprisingly clear. Below are some responses to the question, "Why do you overeat when you want to lose weight?"

"I try to stick to my diet, but always give in to my cravings."

"I can't imagine life without chocolate."

"I'm always sabotaging myself and I don't know why."

"I know I shouldn't eat that stuff, but I can't help myself."

"Each night, I go to the kitchen and pig out — it's like hardwired in me."

"I know I should stop, but I keep eating even after I'm full."

"Once I start, the whole bag is gone."

"I'd go on a diet, but I have no willpower."

"Bread. I love bread. Can't give it up."

"My cravings won't stop. I think this is how an alcoholic feels about liquor."

Underneath most persistent weight problems lie persistent compulsions. In fact without exception, each person I interviewed admitted to suffering a degree of addiction. In academic circles, food addiction is considered rare, but I beg to differ. Food-related addictions are everywhere, though they come in various forms and severities. I think it's not an exaggeration to say that sugar addiction, or processed carb compulsion, if you prefer other terminology, is probably one of the most prevalent health disorders in this country today.

That said, no single program works for everyone and that includes the addiction recovery model. Though I believe addictions and compulsions are pervasive, they are clearly not the only cause of overweight and obesity. Our problems can also arise from endocrine issues, metabolic disorders, neurological disorders, developmental disorders, pregnancy, medication side effects or a simple lack of access to natural foods. And of course, we can have fat-generating carb and insulin vulnerabilities even without suffering from those darn compulsions.

• Savoring a New Normal •

By the new year, I hit about 130 and was on the cusp of entering that previously unattainable zone called normal weight. I couldn't believe it. After more than three decades suffering from a seemingly inalterable case of the chubs, all that fat seemed to evaporate with barely an effort beyond enduring a temporary period of withdrawal. Feeling pretty darn good, I actually added some exercise to my schedule and started practicing gentle yoga from time to time, still without ever breaking a sweat.

From January to April 2011, the weight loss continued, albeit at a slower pace punctuated by various plateaus, until my body settled at a happy 122 pounds. I may not have attained bikini body slimness, but I hit a normal, healthy weight and that was plenty fine by me.

Unlike other diet-induced weight losses, this one felt solid and permanent and I had no problem packing up my old wardrobe into giant plastic bags to give away. Call it addiction transference or just pent-up demand, but in February and March, I shopped like a maniac, happily plucking size 6's off the rack and relishing the fact they, OMG, fit.

More important than my skinny jeans, however, were my sparkling new lab results, including normal blood sugar of 83 mg/dL, normal triglycerides of 49 mg/dL, a normal LDL cholesterol level of 109 mg/dL and a normal HDL of 84 mg/dL. My former health complaints had disappeared. I felt great, had glowing skin, steady energy and a buoyant mood. I felt almost like I had aged ten years in reverse.

After friends asked me to put my newfangled weight loss secrets on paper, I started writing this book. But beyond rehashing my experience, I wanted to understand why this approach worked while others failed, so I dove into the research on nutritional science and biology. It wasn't hard to find the answer: addiction, hormones and biochemistry.

2

The New Way of Weight Loss

◆ ◆ ◆

It turns out my experience was hardly unique. People who adopt the weight loss paradigm based on recovery from addiction and abstinence from sugar and starch are finding remarkable success, even when traditional dieting has failed.

Why is that? The answer seems to be that diet and exercise address the wrong problems. It's not that we're so profoundly gluttonous or lazy. Rather, the problem is we are biologically vulnerable and at the same time, misinformed about the true dangers of certain so-called staples.

Let me explain. Unlike previous generations and certainly unlike any of our more remote ancestors, we are now bombarded with processed, sugary and carbohydrate-rich foods that our bodies are ill-equipped to metabolize. These dense carbohydrates, so plentiful in our modern diet, which include soda, candy, chips, fries, pastries, bread, ice cream, pizza, cookies, juice and pasta, can distort various physiological systems, **sparking cycles of compulsion beyond our conscious control.**

In other words, while real, unprocessed or minimally processed fruits, vegetables, legumes and animal products tend to nourish us without prompting addictions, man-made sugary and carb-rich foods can do just the opposite. Refined sugars, flours and processed foods are so stripped of their fibrous and nutritive content, and sometimes concocted into potent combinations, that they can prompt our Stone Age bodies to react in unusual and often crave-building ways.

To put it bluntly, too many of us are naturally sensitive and artificially addicted. Until we can wrap our heads around that fact, no amount of dieting, exercising or "Let's Move!" types of public health programs will make a real dent in our national health and obesity crises.

So, in the new weight loss paradigm, we seek recovery from addiction without reliance on that ephemeral thing called willpower. We understand that weight loss requires a temporary period of withdrawal from addiction followed by sustained, but undemanding recovery, and not grinding deprivation or hard work. We see refined sugars as potentially addictive drugs and not as just another food ingredient. We understand that starches — found in grains, rice, corn, and potatoes — are long strands of sugar molecules that can also wreak havoc on our blood glucose. We know processed food tampers with our biochemistry and keeps us fat. We pay attention to how our food affects our insulin levels and we don't waste our time counting calories.

It's helpful, though not essential, to understand some of the biochemistry basics behind the new paradigm. So, let's discuss what sugar and starch do to our bodies, how we become addicted to junky or refined foods and why calorie-based diet approaches typically don't work. However, if you're already eager to start, please feel free to skip this part and move on to Chapter 3.

• Not-So-Sweet Sugar •

Who doesn't love a spoonful of sugar? But for many of us, no food ingredient delivers a wallop to our biochemistry like refined sugars do. If you think of sugar as a staple, a necessary ingredient or a natural food with redeeming qualities that you can eat regularly without repercussion, it's time to think again.

Refined sugar is a newcomer to the human diet. Our ancestors started eating it only about 2,000 years ago, a blink of an eye in evolutionary terms, when sugar cane was first cultivated and processed in the Middle East. Sugar crystals made it to Europe more than a thousand years later as returning Crusaders brought small batches of this strange, new substance home with them. For centuries afterward, sugar was regarded as a medicine, a rare luxury item or a once-in-a-lifetime treat.

Sugar consumption began to spread, particularly to the European upper classes who could afford it, only with the advent of massive sugar plantations in the West Indies, Florida and Brazil. The "free" labor of millions of tormented African slaves, toiling under the most brutal conditions imaginable, planted, cut and processed the cane. The human and environmental toll was incalculable. Even today, brutal working conditions and pitiable pay persist on many remaining plantations.

A century ago, Americans consumed less than 40 pounds of refined sugar a year, already a massive quantity by historical standards. Snack food did not exist until the 1920s. And high-fructose corn syrup (HFCS), which replaced table sugar in many sodas, drinks and processed foods, was unknown to the human body until the 1970s.

Yikes! We eat almost 160 pounds of added sugar a year?

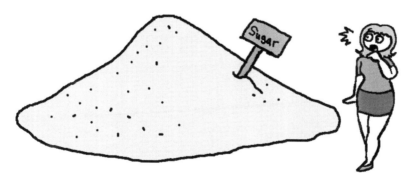

Now we eat an average of 160 pounds of added sugars, including table sugar and HFCS, per person per year. In the span of a few hundred years, sugar went from an almost unknown entity to a ubiquitous ingredient, infusing itself in sodas, juice, cookies, crackers, chips, packaged food, candy, cereal, diet foods, ice cream, dairy products, baked goods, processed meat, condiments and more.

It's important to note that refined sugar is not actually the biggest source of sugar in most of our diets. Many of us get most of our sugar from starches, mainly grains, potatoes, corn and rice. These concentrated carbohydrates break down into sugar during digestion, so metabolically speaking, there's not much difference between a plate of sugar and a slice of wheat bread, even whole wheat bread.

Please keep in mind, that while refined sugar really whomps some people (like me), for others, and I found this to be particularly true with men, the steady starch consumption is the bigger villain. Why that is, I don't know, but the distinction is not terribly significant for weight loss purposes.

A DRUG, NOT A FOOD Increasingly, refined sugar is being understood as a potentially damaging — and addictive — drug and not a nourishing food or even a relatively benign delivery vehicle for empty calories. Think for a moment about how it's made; the result of an intensive, lengthy extraction and purification process. Sugar cane or sugar beets are subjected to a dozen different steps, including crushing, boiling, binding, filtering, evaporation, centrifuging, crystallization, purification, recentrifuging, de-colorization, re-boiling and drying to extract the "active ingredient" of dry, white sucrose crystals. Tell me, is this process how we prepare food or how we extract drugs?

And note the way sugar makes us feel. Unlike foods eaten by our ancestors, sugar exerts a mildly narcotic effect, giving us a "buzz," a "high," a "warm and fuzzy feeling," a "little escape," or a "brain vacation," depending on whom you ask. This offers another sign that sugar can act more like a drug than a food.

Sugar can be devastating to the human body. As a carbohydrate, it exists naturally in fruits and vegetables, of course, but those carbohydrates are usually in low concentrations combined with lots of fiber and vitamins.

After we eat a fruit or vegetable, the food's fiber moderates the entry of glucose into the bloodstream.

But what if there's little or no fiber and a concentrated source of carbohydrate? There's not much to blunt the rapid rush of glucose into the blood.

When we have high blood sugar brought on by food with dense sugars and starches, such as sweets, sodas, bread and pasta, it leads to excess fat that doesn't just sit around our middles like a benign appendage. It also infuses itself in our arteries and organs, setting the groundwork for the variety of chronic diseases we all know too well. Some of the long-term consequences of eating too much sugar and starch include:

- Increased risk of heart disease, stroke, atherosclerosis and high blood pressure

- Increased risk of type 2 diabetes

- Increased risk of certain types of cancer, including breast cancer

- Increased risk of polycystic ovary syndrome

- Elevation of harmful cholesterol, blood sugar, insulin levels and triglycerides

- Increased risk of gout, liver disease and kidney disease

- Increases in hyperactivity, anxiety, depression, drowsiness, concentration difficulties and crankiness

- Tooth decay and gum disease

- Accelerated aging process and weakened immunity

And that's just a partial list. For a more complete list of diseases and conditions caused by eating too much sugar, please visit nutritionist Nancy Appleton's site, www.nancyappleton.com for "141 Reasons Sugar Ruins Your Health."

Sugar by Any Other Name
Is Just as Sweet

When we hear sugar, we may think of sucrose in the form of white crystalline table sugar, but because sugar has so many monikers we are often eating more than we think. My current favorite euphemism found in all sorts of supposed health foods is "evaporated cane juice." Thought you fooled us? Well yeah, you probably did. So here's a list of sugar by another name:

Agave syrup ☐ Barley malt ☐ Beet sugar ☐ Brown sugar
Brown rice syrup ☐ Cane juice ☐ Cane sugar ☐ Caramel
Coconut syrup ☐ Corn syrup ☐ Corn syrup solids
Confectioner's sugar ☐ Carob syrup ☐ Castor sugar
Date sugar ☐ Demerara sugar ☐ Dextran ☐ Dextrose
Diastatic malt ☐ Diastase ☐ Ethyl maltol ☐ Florida crystals
Fructose ☐ Fruit juice ☐ Fruit juice concentrate ☐ Galactose
Glucose ☐ Glucose solids ☐ Golden sugar ☐ Golden syrup
Grape sugar ☐ High-fructose corn syrup ☐ Honey
Icing sugar ☐ Invert sugar ☐ Lactose ☐ Maltodextrin
Malt syrup ☐ Maple syrup ☐ Molasses ☐ Muscovado sugar
Panocha ☐ Raw sugar ☐ Refiner's syrup ☐ Rice syrup
Sorbitol ☐ Sorghum syrup ☐ Sucrose ☐ Treacle
Turbinado sugar ☐ Yellow sugar

It doesn't help that we hear, often from the sugar industry itself, that sugar is "natural." This is true, in the sense it's derived from plants, but so are cocaine and heroin. Natural hardly means "healthy" or "not addictive." Avoid all the items on this list and you'll give your body a fighting chance to recover from its white-stuff addiction.

Furthermore, what seems like moderate sugar intake can add up to a lot of excess weight. Just drinking one can of regular soda a day for one year can put on 15 pounds. For a startling visual representation of how much sugar is contained in many packaged foods (10 cubes of sugar in a single can of regular cola!), please see www.sugarstacks.com. Just looking at how much sugar lurks in our food supply, it's easy to understand how we are suffering autopilot fat accumulation driven by a rate of dense carbohydrate consumption unprecedented in human history.

WHEN BAD ADDICTION HAPPENS TO GOOD PEOPLE While we may have evolved to appreciate the taste of sweetness, our ancestors never had this sort of regular access to cheap starchy carbs and sugar. Wanting the first taste of sugar is natural, but what follows after the addictive cycle starts is not. Evolutionarily speaking, this stuff was not even available or considered possible or imagined. (On the other hand, while those of us with inborn carb sensitivity may not love the way it packs on the pounds, we also have a reason to thank our ancestors for these genes. After all, their more efficient fat storing capabilities made them better able to survive famine so they could pass their genes along to us.)

Not everyone who eats sugar or junky or refined food gets addicted, of course. But depending on our inborn vulnerabilities, many of us do. It's like alcohol — some of us can drink moderate amounts throughout the week without ever developing strong cravings, but others sink into varying degrees of dependence. Let's talk about some of the reasons our junk foods can fuel not just weight gain, but also addictions.

CHANGES IN OUR BRAINS Really fascinating research from the last five years shows that much like street drugs, highly processed food can cause lasting changes in our brains. By disrupting the brain's well-balanced feedback systems, chronic junk food consumption can replace a person's normal ancestral food needs with cravings to seek and ingest more junk food.

First, the function of dopamine, a neurotransmitter associated with pleasure, is disrupted. Junk food produces large and rapid dopamine surges and the brain eventually responds by killing off dopamine receptors and reducing normal dopamine activity. This bullet-ridden dopamine system reduces normal feelings of pleasure and drives the junk food eater to more dopamine-spiking junk to feel "normal" again.

Brain imaging scans have shown that drug addicts and compulsive eaters exhibit the same neurochemical patterns when exposed to the objects of their compulsion. In another study where subjects were shown a milkshake, the same areas of the brain implicated in the urge to use drugs lit up.

Junk food also triggers the release of opioids in a similar, if more subdued manner as drugs like heroin. This also rewires the brain reward circuitry and drives habitual overeating. To make matters worse, sugar also raises levels of the neurotransmitter serotonin (giving us that floaty sense of euphoria), creating yet another source of craving. And should we be surprised to learn that chocolate itself has its own opiate effects?

---

*Like street drugs, highly processed food
can cause lasting changes in our brains.*

THE INSULIN RESPONSE Insulin, the hormone that allows glucose to enter our body's cells, feeds our crazy craving cycle in at least two ways. First, when we eat dense carbs, like bread, soda, pasta or sweets, the pancreas releases a spike of insulin prompting the cells to rapidly absorb the glucose. Low blood sugar follows, leaving us exhausted, cranky and craving more sugar or junk. This is the blood sugar/insulin roller coaster we all know so well, giving us the munchies, the 3 o'clock slump and those nighttime pantry safaris.

But it can get worse. After years of elevated insulin levels due to chronic dense carb consumption, the body can develop a condition known as insulin resistance — the precursor to diabetes — where sugar molecules in the blood

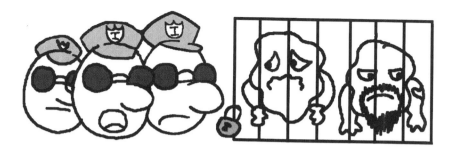

What insulin tells the fat in our fat cells: "As long as we're on duty, you guys are staying locked up in there!" To let the fat escape, we must send layoff notices to our insulin molecules. That means bye-bye to sugar and starch.

can no longer enter the cells to provide energy. The cells are then starved and beg for more glucose, which causes us to feel more hunger and carb craving. This leads to even more carb consumption, which means continuously elevated insulin levels and evermore fat storage coupled with the body's inability to access that stored fat for fuel.

In other words, when we have insulin resistance, we can't burn our own fat for energy and we're always hungry. Ouch. No wonder we fatten up so easily when we ride the carb train.

LEPTIN RESISTANCE Leptin is a hormone that inhibits the appetite, but as we accumulate fat, our sensitivity to leptin decreases, making it more difficult for our bodies to feel full. When the brain can't sense the leptin stored in fat tissues of people with obesity, the brain may sense that the body is starving and kick off feelings of hunger. In other words, the brain needs to be able to sense leptin, but can't do so if it's in storage.

IMMUNE PROBLEMS/INTOLERANCE Some people also suffer what has been called a delayed immune response or intolerance to certain elements of carb-rich foods, especially the gluten found in wheat. Their immune systems create antibodies that may lead to migraines, bloating, heartburn, fatigue and for many affected people, insatiable cravings for the offending foods.

HAVOC WITH GUT FLORA Each of us shelter about 100 trillion microbes in our bodies, most of which appear to exist in a healthy symbiotic relationship with us. They aid our digestion and function in other systems, though we are only just beginning to understand the roles they play. Just like us, our microbes evolved to feed on an ancestral diet free from excessive sugars. Some believe that sugar can wreak havoc with gut flora, leading to problems like intestinal yeast overgrowth. When the yeast get hungry and begin to die, they cause symptoms like nausea, bloating, anxiety, depression and fatigue, prompting cravings for more sugar and starches. So, sugar and carb cravings may, in part, be overpopulated microbes asking for a meal.

• But Wait, There's More •

WEAKENED ADRENAL GLANDS Sugars in the diet weaken the adrenal glands, which sit atop the kidneys, resulting in blood sugar fluctuations. When your adrenal glands are exhausted, you are more likely to consume sugar in large quantities in an attempt to get the energy you need.

PERPETUAL LOW-GRADE MALNOURISHMENT Another factor that may be fortifying your addiction is the possibility you may be eating so many calories of denuded and denatured pseudo-food that in spite of adequate caloric intake, your body continues to hunger for a multitude of macro- and micronutrients.

TASTE BUD FATIGUE Another potential addiction feeder is the concept of taste bud fatigue. By indulging in dense, rich, sweet, salty, highly flavored foods, our taste buds become desensitized to more nutritious, natural, yet perhaps more subtly flavored foods.

With so many biological forces nurturing our addictions (and more being discovered), it's no wonder many of us become powerless over our food. Our sugar and carb consumption really does change us in tangible ways.

• Am I An Addict? •

Our food addictions come in many forms and flavors. No two are exactly alike. For example, there's the woman in her mid-40s who can't get to sleep until she has her nightly nosh of two pieces of chocolate. Or the twenty-something woman who bounces between binging on junk food and temporarily starving herself to lose weight. Then there's the 55-year-old woman with insulin-dependent type 2 diabetes who times her insulin shots to allow for a maximum binge on favorite sweets she hides in a corner of the pantry. Or the 60-year-old man, also with type 2, whose lower legs have been amputated, but who still can't kick his habit of drinking a few cans of cola every day.

And what about your pattern? Is it addiction (that is, suffering compulsions beyond your conscious control) or do you just habitually choose to eat too much? Here are some concepts that can help answer that question:

THE DICTIONARY TEST Dictionaries define the word addiction as an uncontrollable compulsion to repeat a behavior regardless of its consequences. Most of us meet this test with flying colors. How many times have we told ourselves we were going to stop snacking, eating sweets or junk food only to succumb minutes, hours or days later? How many people develop obesity or potentially fatal diseases like type 2 diabetes, yet still can't control their sugar consumption?

THE TWO HUNGERS TEST If you're suffering a food-related addiction, you will have two types of hunger. First is the hunger that comes from our stomach and is directed at nutritious, millennia-old types of food derived from plants and animals subjected to minimal, if any, processing. The second type, a craving coming from that gremlin in our heads, is directed at that processed stuff, like refined sugar, fries, chips or milkshakes.

In other words, when you're foraging through your kitchen for a snack, what's on your mind? Is it salad, an apple, cauliflower, halibut, tofu, broccoli, cottage cheese, eggs, lentils or kale? Or are you craving donuts, cookies, candies, chocolate, pizza, ice cream, soda, pretzels or chips? Are you really hungry? Is your tummy growling or at least feeling empty? Has it been about four to six hours since your last meal? If not, that's the second hunger of addiction talking.

THE SHRINK'S APPROACH Another approach is to look at questions psychologists and psychiatrists use to diagnose Substance Dependence (Diagnostic and Statistical Manual, IV). Only three criteria must be met to warrant this diagnosis.

1. Do you need increased amounts of the substance over time to achieve the same desired effect or feeling?

2. When the substance is stopped, are there physiological and/or psychological withdrawal symptoms? Do you take the substance again to relieve or avoid these symptoms?

3. Do you take more of the substance or take it over a longer period of time than intended?

4. Are persistent attempts at cutting down on the substance unsuccessful?

5. Are you preoccupied with the substance and spending a great deal of time obtaining the substance, using the substance or recovering from its effects?

6. Do you reduce or abandon social, occupational or recreational activities in order to use the substance?

7. Do you continue using the substance despite persistent or recurrent physical and/or psychological problems exacerbated by the substance?

Most people with persistent weight problems have no trouble meeting at least three of these criteria. I met four of them.

And there are others. For example, you can look online for the Yale Food Addiction Scale (www.yaleruddcenter.org), the Overeaters Anonymous quiz (www.oa.org) or the Food Addicts in Recovery Anonymous quiz (www.foodaddicts.org). Specifically for sugar addiction, you might look at author Nancy Appleton's helpful sugar addiction quiz (www.nancyappleton.com).

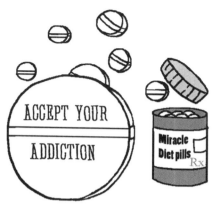

Yes, Dorothy, magic diet pills do exist.

CHOOSE YOUR LABEL If you're not yet ready to commit yourself to a new identity as an addict, I suggest that for at least a few weeks, make-believe you are. See what it's like to think of yourself as powerless over white stuff and eat according to an abstinence-based recovery plan. If after a while you notice a change in your cravings, well-being and control over what you eat, you have finally found something that works, whether or not you loved the term "addict."

But most of us can't bypass our faith in our addictions since that belief lays the very foundation for our recovery. **Without identifying our disease, we cannot seek a cure.** If we were to wait for someone in a white lab coat to formally diagnose us as addicted, we would probably be waiting a very long time and become increasingly debilitated in the interim. Quibbling over semantics — what exactly to call the chronic cravings and compulsions we suffer — is sadly rampant in the ivory towers and only serves as an unproductive distraction from the core cause of recovery. If it's not addiction, then what word should we use? And how much does it really matter?

Let me give you an example of an alternative that works for some people. Some people decide at the outset they have an "allergy" to sugar and flour. They know they have an innate sensitivity triggering cravings and chronic health problems. So just as if they'd been diagnosed with a peanut allergy, it became a no-brainer to lay off their own "allergic" foods. Belief in "addiction" or "allergy" is powerful medicine, and combined with a food plan that restores normal biochemistry, is likely the most effective weight-loss approach available.

Whether we call it addiction, allergy, compulsion, craving, or needing-to-stuff-my-face-with-sugar-bombs-until-I-nearly-pass-out syndrome, it matters little so long as it helps us define our problem and our path toward recovery. Ignore all those in academia and conventional medicine who would have you believe your weight and health problems stem from a "behavior" or "choice." **Your overweight stems from a chemically-induced derangement of your metabolism and is not remotely your fault.**

• The Calories Myth •

How many times have we carefully counted our calories, only to find ourselves miserable, hungry, preoccupied with food and gaining the weight right back after we're done?

There are several reasons mainstream diets don't work very well. First, they allow for and sometimes even promote, quantities of starchy carbs and even sugared foods, which are seen as acceptable as long as they fall under the prescribed calorie limit. In fact, grains and starch are often seen as indispensable to a "healthy diet."

Unfortunately, if the carb addiction is not zapped, the dieter, no matter how rich, smart or beautiful, remains at its mercy and is helpless at keeping snacks and sweets out of her mouth. In other words, an alcoholic can't lick his addiction while allowing himself small thimbles of scotch and daily chugs of beer. His chemistry will not have the chance to return to normal and he will remain within the fortress of his addiction. Same with the dieter.

— — — — — — — — — —

Too many of us are naturally sensitive
and artifically addicted.

— — — — — — — — — —

Consequently, eating even limited amounts of so-called "diet food" — think of those 100-calorie pack cookies, packaged "low-fat" dinners, or a diet

> "When Jill started talking about how (some of us) are like
> alcoholics, and that it's essential that we cut out ALL of it
> (ALL the sugar, ALL the flour, ALL the pasta, ALL the carbs),
> I really started to think about it. I realized that it is easier
> for me (a 'foodaholic') to go cold turkey. I realized that once
> I start eating the sugar and carbs, it becomes like a train out
> of control. I can't have just one cookie!"
>
> ~ Marti R.

brand's chocolate cake — is a very hard way to lose weight. Cutting out the stuff entirely, as with the plan outlined in the next chapter, is much easier.

Second, a conventional diet leaves us hungry and when we're hungry, our metabolisms slow down and our bodies become more efficient at storing fat. Hunger also promotes episodes of binging. Never go hungry while you're trying to lose weight; your biology will ultimately pummel your willpower.

Third, a calorie-counting approach ignores the fat-generating property of excess insulin. A 200-calorie "diet" chocolate shake (packed with forms of sugar) has a vastly different impact on our health and long-term ability to lose weight than a 200-calorie kale salad. Calories are not all created equal.

In sum, if we want long-term recovery and not merely the fleeting state of calorie reduction, it's critical for us to avoid all forms of junk food, no matter how beautifully packaged or what diet program is selling it. Dieting is no substitute for recovery — a nutrition plan means nothing to a junkie.

What We Put in Our Heads Determines What We Put in Our Mouths

I have found that the people who successfully lose weight and keep it off store powerful beliefs in their heads, like these:

- "I'm allergic to the white stuff."
- "I am a drug addict. The only path to recovery is abstinence from my drug."
- "I want to maintain my recovery even more than I want that snack."
- "My body's too sensitive to eat grains."
- "I can't recover from my disease if I eat that."
- "I am an alcoholic with carbs."
- "That's not my food."
- "If we fed monkeys in the zoo the junk I fed myself, I'd be locked up for animal abuse."

On the other hand, the people who can't seem to keep their weight off tend to have conventional thoughts like these:

- "Everything's okay in moderation."
- "It's OK to eat that pizza if I stay within my daily calorie range."
- "They say grains are part of a healthy diet."
- "It's OK to eat sugar as long as I count my total carbs."
- "I'll have the second serving because I can work it off later at the gym."

The depth of our belief in our addiction is directly proportional to our success in losing weight and keeping it off. Just like any addict, when we waver in our belief, we open the door to relapse.

3

What Can
We Eat?

◆ ◆ ◆

As we've seen, effective weight loss begins with the robust repair and normalization of our biochemistry. The good news is that the best medicine to help us accomplish this recalibration is fairly inexpensive, readily available and over-the counter — it goes by the name of real food.

- - - - - - - - - - - -

Easy weight loss hinges on finding
the real biochemical you.

- - - - - - - - - - - -

The food plan offered here is based on my own experience, the stories of others who have recovered and the advice of many outstanding experts. But there's no one perfect, one-size-fits-all food plan. We all have somewhat different sensitivities, trigger foods, blood sugar problems and metabolisms. Don't reach for objective perfection, but use the following fundamentals to experiment a bit and find what works for your particular situation.

• The No's •

Let's start with what we can't eat. Eliminating sugar, white flour, other starches and processed food may sound daunting at first, but once you start down this road, each step becomes easier than the last. That's because (1) our cravings subside; (2) we lose our taste for the stuff; (3) we develop a heightened enjoyment of more satiating real food; (4) we become spoiled by looking better and feeling better; and (5) we rid ourselves of various guilts and obsessions that wasted our time and energy. After a while, there comes a point where we know there's no going back.

NO REFINED SUGARS None. Zero. Zip. The stuff is gross and has been poisoning our bodies and brains. Let it go. Besides, after the weight loss, some of us can tolerate the occasional detour without triggering a full-bore relapse.

NO WHITE FLOUR Again, because its biochemical impact is similar to sugar, white flour cannot be part of our recovery. After a while, you'll think of it as tasteless dust (which it is) and you won't miss it a bit.

Eight great ways to stay addicted!

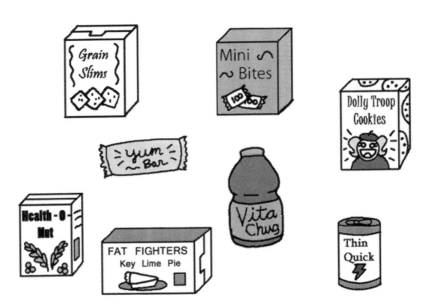

NO OTHER STARCHES Starches support our addictions and increase our insulin levels. I strongly recommend that you stack the deck in your favor and eliminate all other starchy carbohydrates, including rice, potatoes, corn and all other grains, such as whole wheat, rye, oats and barley, during your weight loss period.

Then, after you lose your weight, and assuming you retain a taste for starches, you could carefully experiment with adding back small amounts, maybe some steel-cut oatmeal, sweet potato or brown rice. At that point, you will be in a good position to figure out what starches, if any, your body can tolerate.

NO PACKAGED OR PROCESSED FOOD Packaged or processed food typically contains sugars, including high-fructose corn syrup, as well as trans fats, preservatives, yucky soy products, and food colorings. They have no place in our food plan and that includes all so-called "diet" foods and "diabetic" packaged foods. Those protein bars are just about the same, metabolically speaking, as a candy bar. And those baked goods, desserts and shakes packaged with the logo of calorie-oriented weight loss programs? That stuff tweaks our biochemistry like crazy and is simply not appropriate for anyone serious about recovery from sugar or starch addiction. **If it has a label, it stays off our table.**

NO SUGARED OR HEAVY DRINKS No sodas, fruit juices, commercial fruit smoothies, energy drinks, vitamin drinks, beer, hard liquor, flavored cappuccinos, lattes or milky coffee drinks. Milk is full of sugar, so it's best to save dairy products for meals. After your weight loss, you can carefully experiment with resuming occasional fancy coffee drinks and booze, but for now, they're a no-no.

BE CAREFUL WITH PROCESSED MEATS Steer clear of fatty, salty, processed stuff like hot dogs, fast food burgers and lunch meats. Processed meats often trigger overeating with their high combo of salts and fats, carb-y fillers and unhealthy chemical additives.

NO OTHER TRIGGER FOODS We all can think of other foods that trigger overeating or even binging. They vary person to person, but aside from the carb-y stuff, common ones are nut butters, cheese, bananas, dates, apple sauce, dried fruits, pistachios and other nuts, meat jerkies, wine, diet sodas or sweet tasting marinades. Try to figure out your own triggers and add those to your "no" list.

Some people can sense exactly what foods trigger their cravings or binges, while others aren't so certain. You can find hints in your feelings and behavior. If a food gives you a floaty feeling, a little high or a jolt, it's probably a trigger. And, if you can't have just one or find yourself hungrier after eating some, same there. Or if there's something you just can't resist, even when you're not hungry, bingo. You might consider keeping a food diary to help yourself figure out what special items to put on your "no" list.

• What to Eat •

Our core recovery comes from eliminating sugars, grains, starches and processed foods — and eating a vibrant, colorful array of delicious and nourishing food without ever going hungry or feeling deprived.

Start with food you absolutely love from the following list and fine-tune your plan as you go. Feel super sensitive to all sorts of carbs? Go ahead and try ratcheting up the protein and fats. Dislike salads? Eat cooked veggies instead. Fear the sugar in fruits? Eat a breakfast of fried eggs with sautéed spinach, and forget the bowl of berries. Craving a burger? Sure, but wrap it in lettuce instead of a bun.

Of course, it's impossible to list every decent food option, but this should be plenty to get you going. And be picky. This plan saves so much money (I'm hard pressed to spend more than $6 to $12 a day on food for myself) that we can now afford the very best produce, dairy and meats.

A typical meal will have about 4 ounces, but up to 6 ounces for men (after cooking) of protein, a tablespoon of healthy fats, and the rest of the plate covered with veggies and/or salad. Here's what to eat:

VEGETABLES Broccoli, Brussels sprouts, cabbage, carrots, cauliflower, lettuces, kale, chard, bok choy, green beans, mustard greens, collard greens, beet greens, spinach, green onions, radishes, turnips, beets, string beans, bean sprouts, zucchini and other summer squash, winter squash, tomatoes, artichokes, asparagus, celery, cucumber, eggplant, mushrooms, peppers, seaweed, onions and garlic.

FRUITS Blueberries, blackberries, raspberries, strawberries, cantaloupe, honeydew, other melons, peaches, apples, pears, plums, nectarines, coconut, persimmons, kiwi, cherries, figs, oranges, tangerines and grapefruit.

In moderation: sugary fruits like mangoes, pineapple, bananas, papaya, watermelon, grapes and dried fruit.

PROTEIN Beef, lamb, poultry (chicken, turkey, game hens), fish, seafood, organ meats, eggs. And forget the boneless, skinless stuff — no more dry, tasteless chicken breasts like those you devoured in the bad old days of high-carb, low-fat failed dieting.

Unless you're dairy-sensitive, include dairy products such as cheese, cottage cheese, cream cheese, plain yogurt, kefir, fresh mozzarella and sour cream. Full-fat dairy is preferable, unless you truly prefer lower fat variations.

FATS Olive oil, butter, coconut oil, avocados, avocado oil, olives, bone broth, bacon. Also, the fats naturally present in grass-fed beef.

Dietary fats are essential to our brain function and physiology, so don't succumb to the fat phobia so common in the old weight loss paradigm. Dietary fat, in the absence of inflammation-building foods like sugars and grains, does not, in fact, make us fat. Fats are also quite satiating and unlike starches, will not affect blood glucose levels or spike insulin. Dr. Walter

Willett, chairman of the department of nutrition at the Harvard School of Public Health, puts it bluntly: "[Dietary] fat is not the problem. If Americans could eliminate sugary beverages, potatoes, white bread, pasta, white rice and sugary snacks, we would wipe out almost all the problems we have with weight and diabetes and other metabolic diseases."[1]

But if I can't convince you to eat fats, go ahead and use oil sprays or liquids, such as tomato sauce or broth for cooking. Just avoid industrial seed oils like corn oil, safflower oil, soybean oil and cottonseed oil, as these cause inflammation and can be damaging to your body. I will just hope and pray you eventually give real fat like butter a chance.

LEGUMES Lentils are fine. In moderation: peas and beans, as they tend to contain a lot of starch. Soy products are usually highly processed and can have damaging hormonal and thyroid impacts, so try to avoid them.

STARCHES/GRAIN (The caveat) I realize I told you to avoid eating starch or grain. But some of you just can't get over the "healthy whole grains" myth. So, okay, if you can tolerate them without triggering cravings or unduly elevating your blood sugar, you could try including modest amounts (no more than a total of 4-6 ounces per day) of quinoa, brown rice, sweet potatoes, yams, whole oats, rye, spelt, millet or amaranth. Sweet potatoes and yams would be at the top of the list. Whole wheat, which can have the same sugar impact as white flour while offering little in the way of nutrition, would take last place. Remember, the best way to break the damaging insulin cycle that made us fat is to remove the dense carbs that unduly elevated blood glucose to levels our very sensitive bodies could not tolerate.

To illustrate the sugar content of starchy carbs compared to other carbohydrates, one cup of spaghetti has about 40 grams of carbohydrate, whereas a cup of cooked butternut squash has about 21 grams, a cup of boiled cauliflower 5 grams and a cup of cucumber 2.8 grams. When you eat a salad instead of pasta, you not only eat fewer calories, you keep your insulin levels low and steady. That enables your body to use the glucose and burn fat and it prevents you from feeling hungry just an hour or two later.

[1] Los Angeles Times, "A Reversal on Carbs," December 20, 2010.

NUTS AND SEEDS Almonds, walnuts, cashews, pecans, pine nuts, pistachios, Brazil nuts, sunflower seeds, flax seeds. These can be raw or sprouted, but avoid roasted, salted or flavored nuts and seeds. And no nuts at all if they are among your trigger foods.

EXTRAS Spices, herbs, soy sauce, vinegar, lemon juice, horseradish, hot sauce, mustard, Worcestershire sauce, salad dressing, catsup (in moderation, as it contains sugar), oat bran, salt, pepper.

A special note on salad dressing. I recommend eating a lot of salads — spinach salads, chopped salads, mixed salads, Cobb salads, you name it — so salad dressing is actually an important topic. It's best to make your own, using ingredients like olive oil, vinegar, balsamic vinegar, lemon juice, crushed garlic, mustard, salt and pepper. Commercial dressings often have undesirable ingredients like soybean oil, sugar, high-fructose corn syrup or MSG. But if you have a particular love for a certain commercial salad dressing, I would say okay, if that's what it takes to lure you into eating your veggies.

DRINKS Water, tea, iced tea, coffee, lemon water, broth. You should have no- or at least very low-calorie drinks throughout the day. Vegetable juice and tomato juice are also fine. Just be sure to count them among your vegetable servings.

Many people ask me about diet sodas and diet drinks, like those iced teas I drank during my withdrawal period. My best advice is, if you feel a strong need for them in the short term to help you through the cravings, go ahead. Even now, I often use a small pinch of stevia in my lemon water to take the edge off the bitterness. But given the open questions about the long-term safety of most artificial sweeteners, it's best to avoid or limit them if you can.

Hungry No More

"If I had to characterize my relationship with food in one word, that word would be hungry. Because of my constant hunger, I have battled my weight since I was about 12 years old. I have tried many different diets and successfully lost 17 pounds on Weight Watchers, but the only way I did this was feeling as if I was starving myself for several months.

I developed gestational diabetes with both my pregnancies and since the birth of my son, the diabetes decided to stick around. I have been taking an oral medication to control my blood sugars, but my doctor had to increase my medication because I was becoming more and more insulin resistant.

I always knew that truly eating low-carb would solve my problems, but I never felt focused enough to give it a try until I talked to my friend Jill. I decided to give it a month and see if it could work for me.

Since starting this new way of eating I have noticed two very important things. One, I am hardly ever hungry. I am now positive that my constant hunger was due to constantly eating carbs. The second thing I have noticed is my blood sugars are much more under control. I am still taking my medication, but I am hoping to cut back as my blood sugars continue to stabilize.

I eat mostly eggs, cheeses and other forms of fat and protein, and also plenty of fresh fruit and vegetables. I rarely feel the urge to eat high-carb foods like bread, cereal, rice or potatoes any longer and with my hunger now well under control, I feel much more at peace with food and finally ready to take control of my diabetes."

~ Iesha A.

• Sample Weekly Shopping List •

Here's a sample list of what I buy in a week. Of course, it changes depending on my mood and with the seasons, but this is meant to give you an idea of what your shopping cart may now look like.

PROTEINS A pound or two of chicken thighs with bone and skin, a pound of chicken livers (for chopped liver — don't make fun of me — it's super nutritious and I must say, delish), a pound of beef or fish and a dozen eggs.

DAIRY Some fresh mozzarella, cottage cheese or plain yogurt, preferably goat's milk yogurt.

FRUIT Pears, cantaloupe, grapes, plums and berries.

VEGGIES Mixed greens, cabbage, spinach, cucumbers, cherry tomatoes, squash, onions and mushrooms.

NUTS Almonds and walnuts.

PANTRY STAPLES Sea salt, pepper, garlic, lemons, olive oil, coconut oil, soy sauce, spices, tea, coffee, stevia.

If it has a label, it stays off our table.

At the grocery store, keep to the outside periphery. Avoid the Vortex of Doom of the cereal, bakery, cookie, cracker, chip, juice, soda and ice cream aisles. Also, consider expanding your shopping to alternative sources like produce stands, farmers' markets, local farmers who sell direct, fish markets and specialty butchers. If you want to buy in bulk, Costco often has attractive produce and meats at moderate prices.

Community supported agriculture is also a great way to get high quality, seasonal local produce, dairy and meats, and your bags are usually delivered right to your neighborhood. For more information, see the Local Harvest website at www.localharvest.org/csa.

• Sample Meals •

Ideally, aim for three full meals a day and no snacks, since insulin regulation improves with longer periods between meals and it's easier to resensitize our bodies to hunger. If that doesn't suit you, feel free to have four or five mini-meals, but recalculate portions accordingly. Or have three meals with one or two light snacks like nuts, cheese and fruit.

As they say in Overeaters Anonymous, plan what you eat and eat what you plan. Random, willy-nilly eating made us fat and control over our food helps make us healthy. When we plan our food, we can easily distinguish between the act of feeding ourselves and feeding our compulsions. We may have to dodge some cravings, particularly in the very beginning, but we should never feed ourselves less than what our true hunger demands.

BREAKFAST Feel free to have standards like eggs, bacon, plain yogurt, cottage cheese and fruit, of course. But biologically speaking, there's little reason to stick to so-called "breakfast foods" in the morning. Feel free to add fish, meat or cooked vegetables, which is common in many cultures. Here are some sample breakfasts:

Yogurt *(4 oz plain) with a small sliced pear or berries (4 oz), an egg fried in coconut oil and coffee with milk*

Salmon *(4 oz) with seaweed salad (4 oz), a handful of macadamia nuts and green tea*

Cottage cheese *(4 oz) with cantaloupe (5 oz), 3 slices of bacon and tea*

Two eggs and a small sausage, *sliced persimmon and coffee*

LUNCH AND DINNER As a rule of thumb, try a salad and/or veggies, a protein, plus some fruit and nuts. And don't forget your healthy fats with every meal. Here are some sample meals:

Chopped cabbage salad *with tomatoes, cucumbers, almonds, avocado and lentils. Serve with grilled chicken and half a pear*

Poached salmon *served with spinach salad, tangerines, cashews and avocado*

Chicken breast *cooked with balsamic vinegar and raisins, served with cauliflower in curry and olive oil, and a mixed green salad*

Snapper *cooked in lemon, olive oil and garlic, served with sautéed spinach with pine nuts and an orange*

Baked butternut squash *served with plain yogurt and a chopped salad with garbanzo beans*

Grilled beef *served with braised mixed greens and beet salad*

Grilled chicken *with mixed roasted veggies*

Green salad *with hard-boiled eggs, sliced grapes, walnuts, fava beans and avocado*

Chopped chicken liver *on cucumber slices, served with mixed fruit salad and nuts*

Stir fry *with veggies and beef*

Skirt steak *served with wilted kale and pine nut salad*

Artichoke frittata *served with sliced melon and spinach salad with feta cheese*

Chicken soup *with mixed veggies, including carrots, celery and fava beans*

Grains: Part of a Healthy Diet?

In the new world of weight loss, there's a growing recognition that grains and their derivatives are playing a leading role in the obesity and diabetes epidemics. Some consider the impact of grains even more insidious than the impact of refined sugars.

Grains were not part of our ancestral diet and our bodies did not evolve with them as a principal food source. They are a novelty in the human diet, introduced only about 10,000 years ago in the Middle East. Anglo-Saxons didn't have grains until about 3,000 years ago.

Grains have a special place on our shelves, not because of their nutritional relevance or richness, but because they were more easily stored and transported than other food materials, which helped sustain growing populations in developing communities. No one will dispute the crucial role grains have played in human history and the development of trade and civilization. In addition, refined or "white" flours offered important health benefits through much of history because the refining process eliminated mold and fungus present in the darker unrefined grains.

However, none of this means grains are optimal or even necessary for nutritional reasons. Compared to vegetables, fruits and animal products, grains offer very little nutrition and even contain toxins and antinutrients. Also, millions of us have celiac disease or are sensitive to gluten, the protein found in many grains, including wheat, barley and rye. Gluten increases inflammation and inflammation increases insulin resistance, depresses our immune system and is the basis of many chronic conditions. Grains have also been implicated in gastrointestinal problems and autoimmune disorders.

But don't we need fiber from whole grains to cleanse our gunked-up intestinal tracts, you ask? Certainly not. We can find adequate fiber in non-starchy vegetables and fruits, which we are now eating in abundance And if we need a little extra help, some chopped cabbage salad or psyllium husks can get things moving.

Even assuming you eat grain products for fiber, most of the grains we eat today have little or no fiber. In fact, elimination of fiber from fast food and many processed foods is deliberate, since the presence of fiber shortens shelf life, makes the food difficult to freeze and makes cooking more time-consuming and complex.

So bid adieu to the grains. They tasted bad anyway.

• Recipe Resources •

I am perfectly happy eating a simple meal of simply prepared food without consulting cookbooks. But if you're more of a culinary adventurer than I, there are a zillion books and websites that can help. Here are just a few worth checking out:

About.com.Low-Carb Recipes by Laura Dolson,
www.lowcarbdiets.about.com.

Carb Wars: Sugar is the New Fat by Judy Barnes Baker,
www.carbwarscookbook.com.

Everyday Paleo by Sarah Fragoso,
www.everydaypaleo.com.

The Good Carb Chef, Real Food, Real Easy by George Stella,
www.stellastyle.com.

Healthy Carb Cookbook for Dummies by Jan McCracken,
www.janmccracken.com.

1001 Low-Carb Recipes by Dana Carpender,
www.holdthetoast.com.

Nom Nom Paleo blog,
www.nomnompaleo.com.

The Paleo Diet Cookbook by Loren Cordain,
www.thepaleodiet.com.

The Paleo Solution by Robb Wolf,
www.robbwolf.com.

• The Ultimate No-Brainer Food Plan •

- Almost any salad recipe, but hold the wontons, rice sticks, and croutons and use homemade dressings.

- Almost any meat, fish or poultry recipe, but nothing breaded.

- Almost any non-starchy vegetable or fruit recipe.

When people ask me, "No sugar or starch? What do you eat?" I have to kind of chuckle. I have never eaten such a huge variety of delicious dishes since dropping the boring white stuff.

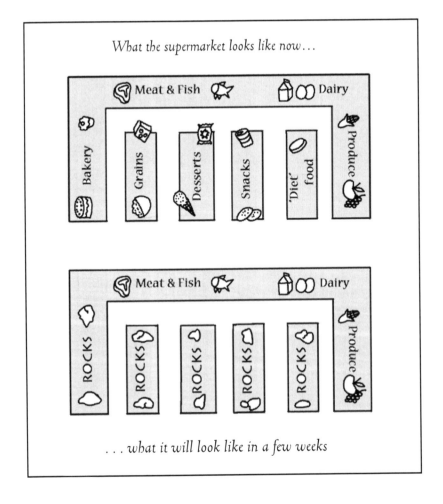

What the supermarket looks like now...

. . . what it will look like in a few weeks

Weathering Withdrawal

◆ ◆ ◆

Withdrawal usually begins six to 24 hours after we stop the sugars and carbs, although some of my friends would say one second afterward. Commonly reported symptoms include craving, fatigue, moodiness, lack of pleasure, confusion, distractedness, anxiety, irritability and discomfort.

Not hugely fun I know, but keep in mind all the wonderful things that are happening in your body. The neurotransmitter system is repairing itself. The gut lining is being replaced. Your immune system is fortifying. Your taste buds are resensitizing. Your thyroid is healing. Cancer cells (which exist in all of us) are starving and dying. Your insulin levels are dropping. Your sensitivity to leptin is reinvigorated. And inflammation throughout your body is dying down.

The good news is that withdrawal tends to get easier each day until ultimately, the symptoms all but vanish. At first our sugar gremlin will screech with cravings, begging us for a fix, but after a while, sometimes just a few days, sometimes a few weeks, that noise fades to merely a whisper.

Because the gremlin at first will not be denied, I recommend that you plan for a supported withdrawal, which could include any of the following:

SUPPORT GROUPS Mutual support groups like Overeaters Anonymous can be a godsend. They are free, run by volunteers and brimming with help, including the availability of sponsors who can help you set up and stick to a food plan. Please note that these groups usually follow the intense 12-step addiction recovery process focusing on emotional, spiritual and physical recovery, so they may not feel right for everybody. But generally speaking, I can't recommend OA and similar groups highly enough. They understood food addictions many decades before clinicians and researchers caught on.

Though admittedly I was more like a fly on the wall than a full participant in any program, I am so grateful for the lessons I learned and the people I met. In the new world of weight loss, there is nothing more powerful than learning directly from others who have walked this road before you.

FIND A PARTNER There's strength in numbers. Find a friend or colleague who shares a similar challenge and act as each other's coaches while you detox.

PODCASTS, BLOGS AND YOUTUBE Stay out of the kitchen and plugged into some fantastic podcasts. For interviews with nutrition, medical and weight loss experts, check out the gold mine at Jimmy Moore's **"Livin' la Vida Low Carb Show"** at www.livinlavidalowcarb.com. To hear narratives by recovering compulsive overeaters/food addicts posted by various **OA groups**, try www.oalaig.org or other OA groups on iTunes. For sound advice from some enlightened licensed nutritionists, listen to **"Dishing up Nutrition,"** at www.weightandwellness.com. For news and updates from the "Paleo" diet perspective, which largely overlaps with our food plan and philosophy, try **"Latest in Paleo"** at www.latestinpaleo.com. And for more on sugar addiction and natural weight loss, listen to **"Diet and Health Today"** with Zoe Harcombe, www.dietandhealthtoday.com.

On YouTube, I recommend University of California, San Francisco

Professor Robert Lustig's lecture about sugar and high-fructose corn syrup called, "Sugar: The Bitter Truth," and from the University of Florida, Nicole Avena, Ph.D. in the video, "Food and Addiction: Sugar Addiction — Proof of Concept." Also, look up Gary Taubes' "Why We Get Fat" IMS Lecture (in eight parts) from August 12, 2010.

Alas, there are too many wonderful blogs, videos, podcasts and websites to list. If you check out the Resources section at the end of this book, you'll find some names of leaders in this field. Search their work online and you'll find a ton of information.

THE ELIXIR OF LIFE Drink, my friend, drink! Instead of noshing when those cravings hit, fill yourself with what I call the Elixir of Life, which is basically water, lemon, and small pinch of stevia, but any citrus-y variation will do. The elixir has lots of benefits. The high dose of vitamin C boosts your immunity and the pectin content reduces hunger. The stevia takes the edge off the sourness and gives a hint of sweetness. Staying hydrated helps keep hunger at bay between meals, so find a bottle to keep at arm's reach. Also, you make it yourself, so it's pretty inexpensive, especially if you have your own lemon tree. If you don't have the good fortune to have access to a trove, go ahead and buy bottled lemon juice or even lime juice, as long as you find it enticing enough.

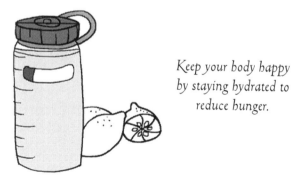

Keep your body happy by staying hydrated to reduce hunger.

PROFESSIONAL HELP Some counselors and therapists who work with drug addiction have tools to help clients through sugar/starch/carb withdrawal. However, I caution against hiring anyone who would psychoanalyze the root of your addiction — you have a chemical problem and not a character defect or a repressed issue involving your mother. Yet, a good therapist can ask you important, probing questions, such as, "Why do you think you can't recover from obesity? Why do you say you can't cope with withdrawal? Why do you say you'll never regain power over your cravings? How many more cupcakes do you need to be happy?"

Nutritionists and dietitians can be helpful too, but they can also be tricky, since they tend not to be well versed about food addictions and can feel obliged to tout party-line mantras like, "everything in moderation" and "grains are part of a healthy diet."

KITCHEN CLEAN-OUT Go through the pantry and toss your junk food and starchy carbs in the garbage or give them away. Tossing excess or unhealthy food is surprisingly difficult for many people — we seem to have a primal urge to hold on to our food stores.

Since the four other members of my family had little interest in participating in my new way of eating, the first few months my kitchen was packed with cereal, bread, cookies, chocolate, pasta and the like. Fortunately, I quickly lost my desire for these goods and realized that my kitchen was basically a microcosm of the real world where, whether we like it or not, we're surrounded by sugar and carbs — at the market, at work, at restaurants, the coffee shop, everywhere. Avoidance at home became something like practice for the carb-saturated world at large.

CLEVER SUBSTITUTES If you feel you can't live without your favorite carbs at first, try some optical illusions to fool your eye, but not your metabolism. Some examples: mashed cauliflower instead of potatoes; baked, stringy eggplant, instead of spaghetti, in marinara sauce; or a small side dish of chopped almonds instead of rice.

PORTION CONTROL Keep in mind that if portion control currently presents a problem, that issue may abate over time. As we eliminate our craved foods, our tendency to overeat diminishes and portion control becomes more natural and less contrived.

HELPFUL MENTAL MANTRAS When cravings hit, it's basically a battle between your head and your "gotta-grab-that-bag-of-chips" gremlin. Give your true self the advantage by storing some of these mantras in your head. They are our primary, indispensable weapons.

- *"I want to maintain my recovery even more than I want that snack."*
- *"My body's too sensitive to eat that."*
- *"That's just my addiction talking."*
- *"When I put my fork down at the end of lunch, I am done eating until dinner time. I will not feed my gremlin."*
- *"I have other ways to fill this need."*
- *"I am a drug addict. The only path to recovery is abstinence from my drug."*
- *"I just need to try to get through the next hour."* (We build our sobriety moment by moment, day by day. We may not be able to deal with 100 cravings at once, but we can certainly deal with one at a time.)
- *"It's so much easier to avoid it entirely than to eat even a little bit."*
- *"I can't recover from my disease if I eat that."*
- *"That dessert is not tempting me, it's tempting my addiction."*
- *"Why am I having seconds? Is it feeding me or my addiction?*
- *"That's not my food."*
- *"The white stuff is Starch Enemy Number One."*
- *"I plan what I eat and I eat what I plan."*
- *"How many more do I need to be happy?"*
- *"I am an alcoholic with sugar."*
- *"I eat what nourishes me and gives me energy and nothing more."*
- *"I need a drink!"* (OK, of the no-calorie variety. No need to start a new addiction!)
- *"The kitchen is closed!"*

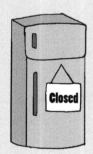

TIPS FOR WITHDRAWAL Kicking sugar addiction gets easier every day, but there will be times you need some extra support and motivation to ease your recovery. When your sugar gremlin rears his ugly head, use these tips to stay on track.

Pair up *Share your newfound quest with a friend — to trade ideas, offer a hand, and maintain momentum.*

Turn on your iPod *Listen to the podcasts listed on page 42. They offer more free advice than you'll know what to do with.*

Stay hydrated *When you have an urge to snack, sip instead. Carry a bottle of lemon water or other natural, sugar-free beverage to keep hunger at bay. (Remember my reliance on diet iced teas in my early days of withdrawal?)*

Toss the junk *Get rid of those sweet and starchy carbs in your pantry so you won't be tempted by foods that did nothing but keep you overweight and addicted. If your family balks, remind them that your health depends on it.*

Reject and replace *When you crave a snack, reach for nuts, fresh fruit or a cheese stick instead of sweets, junk foods and starchy carbs.*

Write and recover *Keep a food journal and note which foods make you feel satisfied and which start your addictive cravings. Eliminate trigger foods from your home, car and office.*

Plan ahead *Tackle parties, potlucks and other social occasions by either bringing food, eating before you go or pre-planning what you will eat. Remind yourself that trigger foods only further your addiction.*

Talk to yourself *Choose one or two self-help mantras that remind you that you are no longer a slave to addiction and are on your way to recovery.*

One and done *If you slip up don't worry, it's just one meal or portion. Be gentle and forgive yourself. Then, get back on the plan.*

Get in bed *If the cravings are killing you, climb into bed and pull up the covers til it passes. Alternative: go to the gym and pretend to exercise.*

That said, some people need ongoing help with portion size. If you're among them, I suggest either using the "hand" method or using a kitchen scale to bring your eyes into synch with your stomach. In the hand method, a meal's protein is about the size of your palm, the vegetables can fill the rest of the plate and the fats — oils, avocado and nuts, for example — would fit into your cupped palm. With the scale, aim for about 4 ounces of protein, but up to 6 ounces for men (cooked), and 6-8 ounces of veggies. Fruit servings should run about 4 ounces. After the weight loss, you can play with upping portion sizes.

Also, if you prefer to count calories as an alternative to portion control, go ahead. But I found very few people who benefitted from counting calories after they eschewed those sugars and starchy carbs.

• Those Nagging Doubts •

Sometimes during the withdrawal phase we'll wonder if it's all worth it, if what we're doing is right or useful or whether we may as well order a pizza and call it a day. Here are some of the common doubts that float through our heads when we get started and some ideas about how to answer them:

"WHY HAVEN'T I HEARD ABOUT THIS BEFORE?" It can feel a little lonely to go through a recovery process while the conventional wisdom is still touting diets and calorie counting. We don't hear much about food addictions from our doctors, the major media or the government.

Doctors who practice conventional medicine do incredible, lifesaving work every day. But generally speaking, they are not well versed in the laws of nutrition or nutritional approaches to treating disease and tend to be constrained by a standard of care that supports a high-carb, calorie-based view of weight loss. Furthermore, the research demonstrating the addictive qualities of hyper-carb foods is relatively recent and the concepts of sugar, carb or other addictions has not yet hit the medical mainstream.

Also, perhaps because the doctors have such little time to spend with patients or because the patients themselves ask for quick fixes, some physicians tend to focus on medication and surgery. If history's any guide, though, not only are diet pills largely ineffective, they can have serious side effects including headaches, high blood pressure, heart attacks, stroke, cancer and death. Bariatric surgery is often cited as the other medical option, but unfortunately, patients who undergo the procedures are often not given the chance to first learn about or recover from their underlying addictions. Many regain the weight they lose or suffer complications.

As for television and other major media, they will likely continue to pussyfoot around the issue. Television and media are terrific and fun, but in the end they're about entertainment and profit and not about addiction education. And perhaps you've noticed that the pharmaceutical and processed food industries spend billions of dollars a year in major media ad campaigns, something that may give even the most well-intentioned producer pause.

As for our government, don't hold your breath. The food industries have some of the strongest lobbies on Capitol Hill and not only do they help control food policy and research, they also receive billions of dollars in subsidies from taxpayers. No, aside from some silly lip service, the government will not make meaningful policy shifts to help us lose our weight any time soon.

"DON'T WE NEED MORE RESEARCH?" The science that has already been published on subjects such as insulin response, dopamine response, opioid response and addiction patterns is more than compelling, but science will continue to evolve and change. No amount of research can ever tell us everything there is to know about the impact of various foods on our infinitely complex physiologies. We will never reach a complete understanding.

Even assuming no studies existed, many of us discovered our addictions long before we knew of any research and we didn't need scientists to tell us what we already knew. In the 1950s, did pack-a-day smokers need research studies to tell them cigarettes were addictive? Were cigarettes not actually addictive until 1,000 different studies could be published? Surely not.

So we can accept and treat our addictions even if we never fully under-stand them. The ultimate authority is our own body. Does removing starchy carbs make us healthier, even if we keep hearing things like, "grains are part of a balanced diet?" Give yourself a few weeks on this recovery plan — your body will give you all the hard evidence you need.

"THIS IS JUST MY BODY TYPE" We tell ourselves, "This is just the way I'm built," when we're 30 or 50 or more pounds overweight. "It's my genetic destiny," we think, as we pinch not just an inch of flesh, but three, four or five. Trouble is, we did not inherit our parents' chubby shapes, **we inherited their sugar and carb sensitivities**, which in our carbohydrate-rich environment, built up our wide tummies and hips.

Fat is not a body type. It's an addiction suit, an insulin suit. A foreign layer that takes a hike when we drop our addictions and, hence, insulin levels.

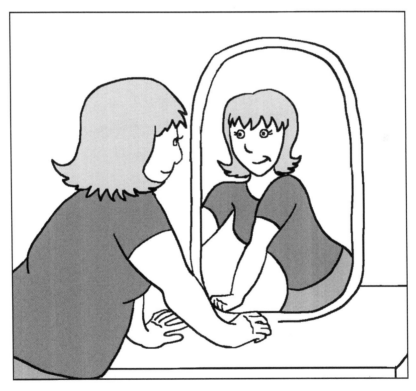

Is your current shape your "body type" or an addiction suit?

Tackling the Real Problem

"Weight issues and dieting have been a constant in my life since I was a teenager. I would try various diet and exercise programs with some success, but eventually the "lost pounds" would creep back on as I struggled to control the other constants in my life — sugar and simple carbs — which I relied on to help me manage stress or provide comfort.

At 46 years of age, I finally came to the realization that I was addicted to sugar and saw how it sabotaged my dieting efforts and over-all health through the years. Since eliminating sugar and simple carbs from my diet last year, I've seen tremendous results not only on the scale, but also with my overall well-being.

In four months, I dropped 30 pounds and my BMI went from overweight at 26.6 to a healthy 20.9. I have more energy throughout the day and no longer suffer the highs and lows of sugar cravings that left me lethargic or cranky from lack of sleep. The new constant in my life is a healthy diet without refined sugar, processed foods and simple carbs!"

~ Denise N.

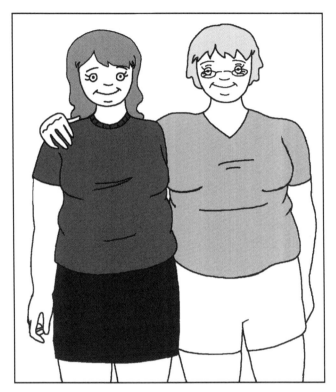

You didn't inherit your mother's hips, you inherited her sugar sensitivity.

Of course we do have different body shapes — wide hips, big boobs, high waists, you name it — but when was the last time we saw a fat skeleton? Body type is, for example, the difference between being 5' 2" and wearing size 2 or 6. It's not the difference between wearing size 6 and size 16. Don't let the body type myth hold you back from lowering your blood sugars and insulin levels to discover the outlines of your real physique.

Not that skinny people are exempt. If you're eating too many sugars or carbs, you're also vulnerable to those chronic diseases, no matter your weight. Better to be well-padded and eating real food, than skinny but running on junk.

"I'M SO STRESSED, I DON'T HAVE TIME FOR THIS" Many people have complained, "I have bigger problems to deal with," or, "I'd lose weight, but I'm too busy/stressed right now." While I'm the first to agree life offers much more urgent challenges than whittling our waist circumference, if you are stuck in a sugar/carb addiction, your body is in perpetual crisis preventing you from being at the top of your game. So, resolving your weight problem can only help you work on all those other goals, right?

Moreover, while weight loss did require oodles of time and energy in the old diet-and-exercise standard, in the new paradigm, nothing about weight loss is hard aside from accepting our addictions and moving past the initial pangs of withdrawal, which for many people are more than bearable.

"LIFE WITHOUT SUGAR OR WHITE FLOUR WILL BE SAD AND BLEAK" If you're like me and like the other former addicts I spoke with, what looks like yummy ice cream today may look like a loathsome, oozing plop of repulsive junk tomorrow. I always believed I loved chocolate chip cookies or a pint of Chunky Monkey. But in reality, it wasn't the food I was after, it was the artificial high it gave me. Once the cravings stopped, I felt only relief to be free of the junk that held sway over me.

Besides, you've already eaten a few hundred donuts, pizzas, cakes, ice cream cones, bags of chips, sodas and supersized fries in your life. How many more do you need to be happy? One, two, a hundred? I'll bet you're starting to wonder if even one more would promote your happiness.

All addictions — whether to drugs, alcohol, gambling or sugar — make our lives smaller, not richer, happier or more enjoyable. When we are enslaved by the constant need for a fix, our lives become increasingly defined by predictable, repetitive conventions and not by creative, intentional living. The bigger our addictions, the smaller our lives.

"BUT MY DIABETES DOC SAYS I SHOULD EAT LOTS OF CARBS" Type 2 diabetes is a serious and potentially deadly disease caused in large part by chronic overconsumption of sugars and starches, which can lead to coronary disease, heart attack, stroke, kidney failure, blindness,

What about Fiber?

While grains have little nutritional value, many people still seem to think we need flours to get enough fiber in our diet. But just as we obtain more nutrition from nonstarchy carbohydrates, we also obtain more fiber. A slice of whole wheat bread with just 2 grams of fiber or a cup of brown rice with 3.5 grams compares poorly with what's offered in the world of fresh veggies and legumes. Here are some examples of fiber content:

Apple, 4g

Broccoli, 1 cup cooked, 5g

Brussels sprouts, 1 cup cooked, 4g

Cabbage, 1 cup raw, 3g

Raspberries, 1/2 cup, 4g

Pear, 5.5g

Lentils, 1/2 cup cooked, 8g

Collard greens, 1 cup cooked, 5g

Avocado, 12g

Flaxseed, 1 Tbsp, 19g

We should aim for 25-30 grams of fiber a day. If we chose whole wheat bread, that would mean 10-15 slices, enough to send our insulin levels to the moon and leave us helplessly lost in Perma-Chub Land. However, eating a salad with a half cup of lentils, chopped cabbage, broccoli, avocado, sliced pear and some flax seeds could easily provide most of the fiber we need for a whole day without spiking insulin and causing fat storage. If you can't get away from the idea of needing bran, you could sprinkle oat bran on your meals or even eat some bran cereal from time to time.

erectile dysfunction, neuropathy (loss of sensation, especially in the feet), gangrene and gastroparesis (slowed emptying of the stomach). It also slows wound healing and increases risk of infection. Given the potential severity of the condition, it's surprising to find so little general awareness about the causes, dangers and treatment of it, even among patients or those who have a family history. Perhaps if we called it what it is, "sugar and starch poisoning syndrome," instead, we'd have better awareness and more targeted and effective low-carb treatment.

Despite the known impacts on blood sugar levels, practitioners have been prescribing fairly carb-heavy diets with toast, potatoes and pasta, for example, even though these foods wreak havoc on already out-of-control blood sugar. This deadly prescription is based on two falsehoods. First, the patronizing belief that diabetes patients are unable to stick to a more healthy low-carb diet. Patients are not given the benefit of the doubt or told how to treat their underlying compulsions/addictions, so they remain in the dark about the very cause of their disease. On top of that is an unfounded worry that a diet high in fat could lead to cardiovascular disease, while it is now clear that high blood sugar and not dietary fat is the culprit.

The good news is these attitudes are changing and, acknowledging research that demonstrates the benefits of low-carb "Paleo" type diets, even the stodgy American Diabetes Association is softening its stance. If you suffer from diabetes or pre-diabetes, I suggest reading *Dr. Bernstein's Diabetes Solution* by Richard K. Bernstein, M.D., which sets the record straight about sugar, carbs and diabetes. Diabetes patients who follow his low-carb recommendations experience better results with some even reversing their disease, than with the standard carb-rich diabetes protocol.

Into a Robust Recovery

❖ ❖ ❖

Once we get through withdrawal, we're 90 percent of the way to recovery. Woo hoo! But there are still a few issues we need to address like exercise, late night eating, snacking, social events and of course, that thing feared by addicts everywhere, the specter of relapse.

THE ROLE OF EXERCISE: IT'S NOT WHAT YOU THINK How many times have you joined a gym and sweated it out regularly only to find a year later you didn't lose a single pound? Exercise has its many benefits, but losing weight is not necessarily one of them. Nevertheless, we should exercise and here are some of the reasons why:

- It's fun or at least it should be.

- It elevates our mood.

- It helps us metabolize glucose and improves our muscles' insulin sensitivity.

- If we're outdoors, we can get some free Vitamin D through sun exposure.

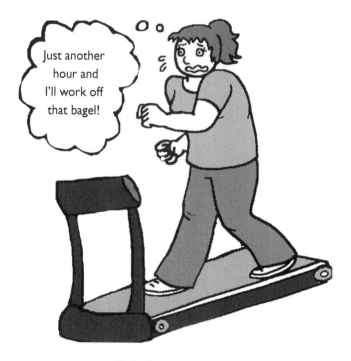

A really bad reason to exercise.

- Depending on your exercise of choice, it can be chummy and social.

- It gives us energy.

- It can help build strength, flexibility, stamina, muscle tone and overall fitness.

- It provides a super distraction to keep us from eating between meals.

But used as an antidote to overeating or to lose weight, exercise is a recipe for frustration. There are multiple reasons for this:

- It's very hard to exercise off a substantial amount of excess calories. For example, you'd have to run for 45 minutes just to burn off a mocha from Starbucks or walk four-and-a-half hours to burn off a Big Mac.

- Exercise can spike your appetite, which invites opportunities for the addiction to re-exert itself.

- If you are exercising to compensate for overeating, you may be in a cycle of exercise bulimia and not addressing the root cause of your problem.

- If you take a break from your exercise program and your addiction remains intact, the inevitable ballooning ensues.

- If you're significantly overweight or of a certain age, strenuous exercise may be more likely to land you in the orthopedist's office than in size 6 jeans.

I know we see a lot of sweating and grunting on weight loss reality shows, but understand that colorful obstacle courses make for better television than watching people not eating sugar and flour. And certain major advertisers might be a tad offended by a suggestion that contestants swear off packaged food and snacks for all eternity.

Please do a thousand push-ups and swim a hundred laps if that's what makes you happy. But for weight loss purposes, moderate exercise like tai chi or walking is usually plenty to get the blood flowing. Say goodbye to those days when we exercised out of guilt or the dark feeling we wouldn't fit into our favorite outfit unless we burned some serious calories. No gain, no pain is a myth. Let's get over it.

• Coping with Real Life •

THE KITCHEN IS CLOSED Sleeping on a full stomach is a great way to gain weight, suffer all sorts of gastrointestinal problems and have impaired zzz's. In my experience, it also triggers morning cravings. We do not need extra energy to sleep and in any event, our bodies' natural rhythms and hormone cycles remove appetite during the night. Moreover, a sustained period of not eating is instrumental in lowering overall insulin levels, which will help with weight loss.

At about 6 p.m. (7 p.m. in the summer), I consider my kitchen closed, and generally refrain from another bite. That said, some people like or need to eat later at night. See what works for you, but if you truly want to burn fat,

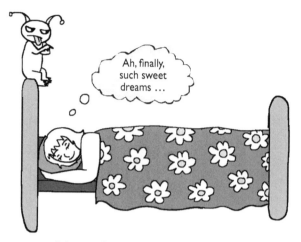

A light tummy while you sleep and away the sugar gremlin shall creep.

it's critical to end or limit late night eating and sleep with very little or no food in your stomach.

RETHINK SNACKS Generally speaking, snacks feed our addictions while meals feed us. After all, when we say, "snacks," doesn't that just mean, "excess stuff we put in our mouths for recreation?" Recovery means the end of recreational eating. So, if you must eat between meals, put those foods into your food plan and do your best to avoid all that impulsive noshing, which got you into trouble in the first place.

PACK UP LEFTOVERS If you have problems with portion control, bring food containers to restaurants knowing you may be doggy bagging half your dish. If you have leftovers after a home-cooked meal, put them in a container pronto and don't even think about doing the piecemeal nosh on them.

COOKING FOR YOU AND YOUR FAMILY People often asked how I could follow this food plan while others in my family remained faithful white-stuff eaters. The answer is, it only took me five or ten minutes to prepare most of my meals, since I took the "simple food, simply prepared" route. Usually, I chopped veggies and stir-fried, baked, pan-roasted or turned them into salad. Often, I would cook enough beef, chicken or fish at once for multiple meals. It truly was easy.

I would like to stand on a soapbox and lecture piously about how I got all my kids to eat my way, but mine are on the extreme end of the picky spectrum and it's an issue I'm still working on. Fortunately, my once skeptical husband joined in the white-food-free lifestyle after just a few months without my having to nag or prod. Well, maybe I did nag a little, but who needs much rhetoric when your own transformation serves as a silent billboard?

DINNER PARTIES, BIRTHDAY PARTIES AND POTLUCKS Ah, temptations galore. Those biscuits, cupcakes, casseroles and nachos probably won't have much appeal anymore, but if there's not much of an alternative, you may be tempted to dig in. So, you have three choices. First, pick at your food. That's right. Just like your mother told you not to do. If the hors d'œuvre is tomato bruschetta, just eat the tomatoes, but leave the bread. If the barbeque is all about hamburgers, eat one wrapped in lettuce or atop a salad and ditch the bun. Second, you could bring your own food. Except at more formal functions, I do this with some frequency and in this day and age of specialty diets, nobody thinks I'm weird. Third, eat ahead of time. Have a dinner planned with friends at 9 p.m? Eat your meal beforehand, but join them at the table for sporting conversation and drinks.

But what if you're throwing a party? You have two choices. Either serve the conventional stuff, but just don't eat it yourself, or try your hand at serving your type of food. We have done both and the results were hardly what I expected. Our after-dinner holiday party featured a table laden with the usual holiday cakes, cookies and chocolates, but our guests seemed more interested in the crudités and cheeses. In fact, a lot of the chatter turned to the subject of how few of us were still eating sugar. And at a recent Paleo-style dinner party, our guests raved about the brisket, mixed vegetables, chopped liver, salad and fruit dessert. No one seemed to miss sugar or starch for a moment.

For appetizers, instead of crackers, put your toppings on sliced cucumber, apple, pear, peach, endive, carrot or celery. For the main course, if you serve a festively prepared meat, a colorful salad and a side of cooked vegetables, no one's going to be asking, "Where's the fettuccine Alfredo?" For dessert, try a glorious tray of fruits, nuts, cheeses and dates — a dream feast — and your guests will leave feeling nourished and satiated, not groggy and engorged.

Life-Changing Energy

"I'm a formerly thin person who slowly gained weight over the past decade or so. Like most people of a certain age, I lost small amounts of weight (numerous times!) using the 'exercise more, eat less' theory, but eventually the weight would creep back because no matter what approach I tried, I felt constantly hungry.

Then I realized I had a problem with sugar and starch, and that my intolerance grew and grew with each step closer to middle age. The withdrawal was not easy at first, but when I began restricting the sugar and starch in my diet, I stopped feeling so hungry and realized this was a way of eating I could stick with. I do not have more willpower than before — I simply have less hunger.

I now have fewer headaches, less joint pain, fewer allergies and more energy. The unexpected result from a low-carb diet is that it completely changed my relationship with food. I used to need to eat small amounts of carbs every few hours.

The most important benefit is having the freedom to leave the house, go to school (I went back to college in my 50s, but thanks to my new way of eating, I have energy to match my much younger classmates) or go about my day without worrying where I will be getting my next 'fix.' It has truly changed my life. The only 'negative' side effect is that my friends are tired of me talking about how easy it was to lose weight!"

~ Jen M.

NAVIGATING THE WORKPLACE At work, think like a construction worker and bring your lunch bucket. You'll have wonderful food and save a lot of money, too. For meetings and office parties, in the event you're wary of bringing up the subject of your sugar addiction, you can do the old quietly-pick-at-your-food trick or cite a food allergy or analogous condition such as gluten intolerance (which, frankly, many of us seem to have). In any event, if you eat the buffet salad, but pass on the sub sandwich, it's likely no one will notice. Of course, when you drop 20 or 30 or more pounds people will begin to ask questions, which I see as a good thing, since some things you just can't hide.

EATING OUT In the beginning, I feared going to restaurants and would first go online to make sure their menus had at least a dish or two that aligned with my food plan. Fortunately, I found my kind of food at most places, even if it meant sometimes giving the waiter specific instructions like, "I'll have the salad, but with the extra chicken and no croutons, please." I went to a wonderful Vietnamese restaurant recently and ordered beef noodle soup adding, "But hold the noodles and double the vegetables, please." Not a problem.

BE PATIENT WITH WEIGHT FLUCTUATIONS Your weight will steadily decline, though in a nonlinear fashion. At first, the weight comes off fast; two pounds a week is common. As we near the finish line, the pace slows considerably to perhaps two-to-three pounds a month. And along the way, we hit plateaus and even some small gains. This can happen for several reasons. We often gain muscle as we lose fat, resulting in stable weight, but shrinking measurements. Our weight can also be influenced by a buildup of water, waste products or for us gals, that premenstrual puffing. So, don't sweat the little ups and downs and plateaus. We're not in a race to see who gets skinniest the fastest.

Just the other week, in fact, after coasting along at a stable 122 pounds, I put on three pounds. Yikes? No, that's just what happens when you have four dinner parties in a row and eat and drink a little too much a little too late at night. Once I resumed my regular pattern, the weight slid back off. Hardly a cause for alarm.

CHEAT CREEP AND HAPPY FAT It seems that for many of us, even those of us who remain sworn off sugar and grains, strict adherence to our food plan does fall victim to a bit of cheat creep after a while. We may start nabbing a few late-night handfuls of nuts or munching an extra cup of fruit after breakfast or eating some of our kid's leftover steak at dinner. But as long as we stay away from the sugary or starchy stuff, does it matter a whole lot? I think the answer varies from person to person, but for most of us, it's no big deal and not necessarily a launch down the slippery slope.

I tend to think along the lines of my friend Jen M., the 50-something college student who seemed to turn back her physical clock after she went low-carb. At size 4, she's hardly what anyone could possibly call overweight, yet, under her teeny jeans lies (gasp!) a layer of pinch-an-inch flesh. It's what she calls her "happy fat," that quantum of cushioning she's happy to live with in exchange for not slavishly adhering to a particular strict portion-controlled food plan and not kicking herself for every little indiscretion. In other words, she'd much rather be a bit sloppy at size 4 than obsessive and miserable at size 2. And I'm with her on that. At my height, I could easily be lighter than 122 pounds, but the way I see it, I'm plenty healthy and energetic, happily free from sugar addiction and would rather eat dirt than become one of those bony obsesso-maniacs. Militance is useful (indispensable) during withdrawal and weight loss, but afterward, play a little.

RESTOCK YOUR CLOSET, BUT PATIENTLY Ah, the subject that tops many a weight loss agenda. Buying a new wardrobe for your new body can be super fun, but I would caution against rushing into it. When I lost my first 20 pounds and hit about 135, I thought there was no way my body was going to get much smaller, so I went a-hopping to the shopping. Oops. Just a few months later I had lost more weight and ended up giving lots of those lovely new clothes away.

We can't tell ahead of time exactly where our body weight and size will settle once we find our biochemical equilibrium. So, I suggest you save your money until your body stabilizes because you may be surprised just how small you'll turn out to be.

HOW DO YOU KEEP IT OFF? Because yo-yo dieting is so common, people are always surprised to see me maintaining my weight loss. I get asked a lot about my "maintenance plan." I answer I have no such plan because once you're not addicted to the white stuff and loving the joys of real food, it's almost impossible to put the weight back on. With my normalized insulin levels and my neurotransmitters back to their calm and measured feedback, I eat lots and lots of healthy food, never go hungry and have lost the overlay of cravings that drive so many dieters back into their old wardrobes.

RELAPSE AND THE JOYS OF IMPERFECT ABSTINENCE As they say, once an addict, always an addict. It's true with drugs, alcohol, smoking and it can be true with our trigger foods, too. So, keeping the weight off depends on exactly what the recovering alcoholics and drug addicts also do: staying abstinent and staying sober.

Most of the time you'll feel solid and confident in your recovery. But there will be days when you feel a bit like a tinderbox, vulnerable to exploding at the merest glimpse of a hot fudge sundae. If cravings and temptations are getting the best of you, I would advise a visit, and pronto, to a support group. Research in drug and alcohol addiction shows that support groups offer the most effective sobriety maintenance support available.

At the same time, no one is perfect and depending on your body's sensitivities, your abstinence need not be perfect either. The way I look at it, my core abstinence is steering clear of sugar and grains. I don't tamper with that, at least not much. But if I venture a bit into the starches from time to time or have some honey in my lemon water, no harm done since small amounts of those foods no longer trigger my cravings.

Straying off course can also provide a valuable learning experience. At a restaurant with my son one evening, I nabbed one of his heavily battered chicken tenders for a munch, but shortly afterwards it felt like a glob of glue had settled in my abdomen. So, my little indiscretion taught me I should indeed continue to steer clear of flour.

After a few months feeling shipshape without sugar and starch, you may feel confident enough to test out some of those foods you had eliminated, too. Dabble in small portions and wait a full 24 hours to see how your body handles it. If it's your birthday and you feel the world will end without a bite of cake, well, what can you do? But try just a bite, which after all, is just as tasty as the whole piece. The only difference is that the whole piece will drug you with that woozy, buzzy feeling and do we really want to revisit that?

And if we fall into a relapse, then what? Well, there's no shame in being an addict and there's no shame in relapse either. It's not our fault or anyone's fault we have this little problem and are susceptible to tumbling back into the void. But recovery, should we choose it, is our right. And that goes for multiple recoveries, too.

While we addicts can never fully lick our addictions, we can certainly reach a point of sustained and happy recovery. When we stick to the principles of the new world of weight loss, we can reach 99 percent normal and feel forever ecstatically imperfect.

◆ You Can Do This! ◆

So at long last you have learned the missing piece to your weight-loss puzzle. Congratulations, your new life is just one moment away.

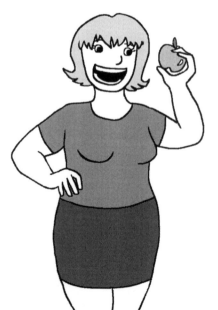

With the sugar gremlin banished, we finally regain control over what we eat.

A Foodaholic Changes Her Ways

"The evening I talked with Jill at a holiday party was a real eye-opener. I have always known that in order to lose weight, I need to control my intake of sweets, carbs, calories, blah, blah, blah. I've done Weight Watchers with some success, but tended to gain the weight back. I have lost weight on my own and I know the drill, but have always felt I was denying myself for a limited amount of time while 'on the diet.'

However, when Jill started talking about how (some of us) are like alcoholics and that it's essential that we cut out ALL of it (ALL the sugar, ALL the flour, ALL the pasta, ALL the carbs), I really started to think about it. I realized that it is easier for me (a 'foodaholic') to go cold turkey. I realized that once I start eating the sugar and carbs, it becomes like a train out of control. I can't have just one cookie!

This time, I'm not thinking of my new way of eating as something that I will do for a certain amount of time. I am thinking of it as my new life. In a way, this is very liberating.

The weight loss was fast at first (about 10 pounds in the first month!) probably because it was such a change for me. Now my body is adjusting more slowly and I'm at normal weight.

The idea that there are specific foods that I just don't touch makes it much easier for me. I have a new attitude about eating and I can truly say I don't miss some of my former favorite foods.

Thank you for inspiring me to make this change … and to change my life!"

~ Marti R.

Appendix A
• Frequently Asked Questions •

How could I possibly give up something as common as sugar?

We are so accustomed to think of refined sugar as a mere "ingredient" with "empty calories" instead of an unnaturally potent substance with profound and addictive physiological effects, that we underestimate its impact on our bodies and behaviors. Living in a world that largely denies the existence of something as manifestly obvious as sugar addiction can make quitting, even for the most die hard anti-sugar advocates among us, especially tough.

So, we give up sugar by conjuring the internal fortitude to defy conventional wisdom, risking the raised eyebrows of our not-yet-fully-informed friends and family, and fully accepting our addiction to the white stuff. Yes, the dope may now spill into every corner of the modern world, but know that for more than 99 percent of human history, not a single human ingested so much as a single cube of refined sucrose or drop of HFCS. Eating sugar is an unnatural act and don't let its ubiquity fool you into thinking it's a normal part of any diet.

There are no such things as empty calories. In fact, the high calorie content of sugar and junk foods are the very least of their evils. This stuff reshuffles our internal chemical architecture and, for those of us with sensitivities, permanently changes the way we respond to food.

I don't feel full unless I have starch at a meal like rice or bread.

Starches are basically long-chain sugars, so when we say starch, we pretty much mean sugar. But do we seek a feeling of "fullness" or rather a feeling of a slight sugar stupor, which is rather distinct from feeling nourished and sated? When a meal of fresh veggies and fish, served with oils, fruits and nuts, feels insufficient without a baguette, what is it about the bread we need? Particularly when it adds nothing of value to our gloriously nutritious and tasty meal? If you're an athlete or laborer who could use some extra blood sugar, that's one thing, but for the rest of us, ponder why inducing a mini food coma should be necessary to round out a meal.

Some diet plans advise a cheat day where you eat whatever you want. Why are you opposed to that?

It's a terrible idea for a sugar addict. Would you tell an alcoholic, "Stay sober for six days and then on the seventh, have at it!" No, because such advice would simply re-immerse him in his addiction and kick-start the same old cycle. It's the same with us.

But can I cheat, ever?

Sure, if you can do so and remain healthy and in control. Here are some ideas: Have some extra dried fruit and nuts, slather some honey atop Greek yogurt, sneak a spoonful of sunflower butter, grab a bag of your favorite beef jerky, have an extra glass of wine with some pungent cheese, eat the whole darn papaya. But beware of cheating with the white stuff — you don't want to go down that slippery slope. Also, please save your cheats and experiments until you've finished with the process of losing weight.

I have no time to cook. How could I follow a plan that allows for no processed or packaged food?

Well, for the past several thousand generations, food preparation took hours every day, but today, we — and this admittedly includes me — complain if a meal prep takes just five or ten minutes. Most everyone is able to prepare simple, tasty meals with minimal effort — salads, stir-frys, cooked veggies, poached fish, sautéed skirt steak, fried eggs or fresh fruit with plain yogurt. You can prepare several meals at once, cutting prep time even further. I estimate I spend only about 20 minutes a day on food prep for myself.

Remember when you learned to ride a bike? It seemed so daunting at first and those handlebars shook like crazy. Feeding yourself this new way is the same. It's a little creaky and challenging at first, but then it becomes so smooth and automatic, you stop thinking about it.

I can't believe that refined sugar is as addictive as drugs.

While of course no one would say sugar crystals hijack our neurotransmitter systems with the same powerful force as, for example, a methamphetamine drug, sugar addiction is so multifold, involving so many physiological systems, that it wraps us up with not just one, but several sticky tentacles. In other words, what it lacks in neurochemical power (and remember, sugar addiction does involve the same neuro-chemical pathways as drug addiction), it makes up in multidimensionality. Sugar creates unnatural imbalances in our neurological systems, hormone systems, immune systems and gut flora systems, to name a few. I was not surprised to hear one of my interviewees say, "Quitting smoking was easy compared to giving up sugar."

Can't I give up sugar without also giving up starches and grains?

If you don't cut the starch you won't lose much weight or you'll lose it more slowly and with more of a struggle, because you're continuing to feed your body lots of long-chain sugars. I suggest giving up grains, even the supposedly healthy whole grains, because they create inflammation, irritation, addiction and allergy in so many people. However, if you feel strongly that you must have starches, I would recommend sweet potatoes, brown rice or perhaps some steel-cut oats.

But don't we need grains to feed the world?

In the short term, probably yes. But in the long run, intensive grain agriculture can be environmentally devastating and lead to the desertification of landscapes and famine. The fertile crescent of the Middle East became arid and dry after the early civilizations adopted grain agriculture. The location considered by researchers to be the once-verdant site of the Garden of Eden in Turkey is now a scrappy hardscape, made so by early agricultural practices that depleted topsoil. Here in the U.S., Midwestern topsoil is being depleted at an alarming rate by aggressive grain-based monoculture.

Don't we crave sugar for evolutionary reasons to avoid starvation?

We evolved to eat real food from the ground or derived from animals and to hunger for what nourishes us, not to be enslaved by cravings for cheap, modern, genetically modified crud that makes us sick. Let's not blame evolution for the perils of modern food.

Is it important to avoid genetically modified food on this plan?

The point is somewhat moot because none of the major GMO crops are included in our plan. Those major crops are sugar beets (sugar), soybeans (soybeans, soybean oil), corn (corn oil, corn syrup, high-fructose corn syrup), cotton (cottonseed oil) and canola (canola oil). However, we do eat them indirectly through conventionally raised animal products, since those animals grow on GMO feeds. If you want to avoid the GMO food chain, choose organic grass-fed beef, organic free-range chicken and wild seafood.

Isn't dark chocolate an antioxidant?

Cocoa is bitter and unpalatable without added sugar. Chocolate as we know it, does not exist without gobs of added sugar. If you want to minimize oxidative stress on your body, stick to a sugar-, starch- and grain-free diet.

Does it always take three weeks to get through withdrawal?

Most people get through the worst of it in about three to five days. Then the cravings, lethargy, shakiness, headaches, crankiness and fog continue to recede over another week or two or three. It varies person to person.

My doctor says I should just eat less and move more.

How many people do you know who actually lose weight that way? How many times have you lost weight that way, only to gain it right back and then some? Permanent weight loss comes from normalizing our biochemistry, not from caloric restriction or shaking our bootie. That means eliminating stuff alien to our bodies' innate metabolisms — refined sugar, white flour and processed food — without making ourselves go hungry or inflicting the self-punishment of chronic cardio. We don't get fat because we eat too much — we get fat because we have been eating the wrong stuff.

Can't I just go straight to a Paleo or low-carb diet? Do I have to do this addiction stuff?

If you can go straight to a healthy eating program like Paleo or low-carb without the physical-mental process of undergoing addiction recovery, more power to you. That said, I've found that for whatever reason, men generally have an easier time going straight to a diet phase than women do.

Doesn't eating fat make you fat?

Dietary fat is vital to human health, brain function and effective weight loss. In the absence of sugars and starches, dietary fat will not make you fat. The only reason I include nonfat and lowfat choices on the food list is because I realized early on that selling the addiction story was easy compared to selling the fat-is-good-for-you story.

I know I need support to recover, but I'm not crazy about Overeaters Anonymous or twelve-step programs. What else do you recommend?

It would be wonderful to see new sugar addiction support groups that entertain topics like food addiction research, basic biochemistry, food history and meal planning, while also offering traditional sharing and peer mentoring. I hope we'll see things like this cropping up. In the meantime, don't shy away from OA, which offers marvelous support. Some nutritionist and dietitians do hold nutrition classes and discussion groups, so ask around.

I seem to have plateaued. What can I do to shed the last ten pounds?

The plan I advocate is about good health and peace of mind, not about runway-model skinniness. If you want to get very lean, however, you can ramp up the strength training and go easy on dairy, fruit and nuts. Also, cut out nighttime eating and snacks.

My big problem is eating at night. How do you stop at 6 or 7 p.m?

See what happens when your sugar compulsions subside. You may be surprised to find you lose late-night munchies, not to mention straight-out-of-bed morning sugar cravings. Diving into bed early, if feasible, will help.

I'm a chocoholic, but I take a statin to lower my cholesterol. Shouldn't that be okay?

Would you break your own leg, then rationalize it by saying you could always buy a splint?

What's your take on artificial sweeteners?

I think they could be useful during withdrawal, but I don't recommend them for long-term use. The good news is you will lose your taste for them over time.

Why is willpower not enough?

Sugar addiction is a chemical process that places our eating habits beyond our conscious control. Willpower means nothing to a junkie.

I'm an emotional overeater, but I wouldn't call myself an addict. Don't I just need to deal with my emotional triggers?

In a word, no. What some people call "emotional eating" is wholly dependent on the preexistence of an underlying physical compulsion caused by an underlying chemical disequilibrium. Moreover, it's not so much that we eat because we're depressed, as we become depressed because we eat sad-making sugared and processed foods.

I've done great so far, but how can I manage through the holidays?

Modern holidays are blood sugar disaster zones. Defend your home against the choco-industrial complex and redefine your celebrations to include only nutritious and delicious whole foods. I have a secret plan to turn October 30 (get it? the day before we shovel mountains of sugar into our innocent children) into Sugar Addiction Awareness Day, so maybe you can channel some of your holiday energies my way and help me with that!

Appendix B
• Lightbulb Moments: Two Trigger Talks •

Sometimes a frank and probing discussion is all it takes to nudge us toward clarity about the roots of our food and weight problems. These "trigger talks" can be remarkably helpful in lifting the fog from our thinking about weight loss and kick-starting the recovery process. Here are two recent talks I had with colleagues, edited for length and clarity.

Try talking with your own friends about their food issues. While being supportive and nonjudgmental, you may be able to help each other gain focus about what is really sabotaging your weight loss efforts.

Monica O., 36, is a San Francisco Bay Area writer and a mother who has had high blood pressure, as well as weight and digestive issues, since her 20s. At the time of our conversation, she weighed 190 pounds and wanted to lose 50 pounds to reach her normal weight.

Can you tell me a little about your weight problems and what you've tried in the past?

I was a heavy kid from the time I was probably in my early teens, even though I've been pretty athletic all my life. Since my 20s, I've been battling my weight with various diets. I've done Weight Watchers, Jenny Craig, weight loss shakes, Medifast, vitamin B-12 shots, low-calorie, low-carb, and pregnancy hormone shots, which I hated. With all of them, you can lose weight for a little while — the most I've lost was about 30 pounds — and then something happens and I just quit and put the weight back on, plus five to ten more pounds each time. It's been a good, solid 15-year battle to get the weight down and get healthier. But now, I'm the second heaviest weight I've ever been.

The most success I've had was when a naturopathic doctor put me on a low-carb Atkins-like diet, mainly restricted to highly cooked vegetables and meat for six weeks. Not just for my weight, but for my gut to heal and not work as hard. Literally, no caffeine, no dairy, no sugar, no starch, no fruit, but I did reintroduce raw vegetables after two weeks. I lost 30 pounds, my blood pressure improved and I felt great. My hair was shiny, my skin was perfect and my normal clothes fit again. The first week was brutal, though. I was a raving bitch. I think I probably should have gone somewhere by myself. I had no energy for at least seven days.

Did it occur to you then, that you might have been going through a sugar and carb withdrawal?

Well, the doctor called it withdrawal because of starving the intestinal yeast, not from an addiction perspective.

Did you feel malnourished on the meat and vegetable diet? Why did you end it?

I felt handcuffed by a lack of variety. I'm a picky eater. Meat, broccoli and cauliflower every day — it was monotonous. Also, the thing for me is the time. My husband has food allergies — no chicken or shellfish — and my daughter is a picky eater. It gets hard and it gets boring. It was hard for me to sustain cooking and shopping for the family when there were complaints and battles all the time.

After six weeks on that low-carb diet, then what?

I went back to how I ate before and gained back 20 pounds in two weeks. I get out of control very easily. It's unsustainable for me to eat that restrictive of a diet.

What did you miss?

I'm not a huge bread eater, but I missed fruit a lot. I remember in my doctor's office almost crying that I couldn't eat nectarines and watermelon, and coffee drinks, too. Vanilla lattes, caramel mochas. I would start my day with a sugared coffee drink. I have a total sweet tooth. I like a cupcake at birthdays or with friends and I loved to make cookies every other week. So, I missed that.

Now, how would you describe how you eat?

I'm generally a healthy eater. For breakfast, usually a Greek yogurt parfait with granola and fruit or a scramble with some bacon or sausage. I love hot sauce on that and coffee. I try to cut back on sugar and I drink a ton of water, 60 or more ounces a day. I have lunch around 11:30 or 12 and it's kind of a crapshoot — a BLT, a taco salad — but I try to have a vegetable or meat and a whole fruit like an apple or an orange. Between 2 and 3 o'clock, I need chocolate. I don't even crave alcohol the way I need chocolate. So, I try to combat that with fruit, an orange.

When you battle against your daily chocolate craving, do you win?

Unfortunately in the office environment, people think they are being nice and have chocolates out on their desks. I can usually stave it off by having the fruit and just one or two Hershey's Kisses or whatever. But there are some days I cannot win.

So, do you have chocolate every day?

About 80 percent of the time, yes.

Why do you reach for it?

Because in the morning, I gave my body white sugar and it's been six-to-eight hours, and it needs its fix. I don't have an addictive personality, so I don't know what it's like to absolutely have to have something like an alcoholic or a drug addict, but I can liken it to an addiction because I didn't need it before. I know what it's like to be off the sugar, so I can compare.

You used interesting language — "it," referring to your body, wanting the chocolate and not "I" who wanted the chocolate.

Well, if you were to ask me, "What's your favorite treat?" I would not say chocolate. So that's the funny thing. But if you ask, "What do I like?" I would have a caramel cupcake or my grandma's berry pie. I wouldn't say I wanted a candy bar.

But it's still sugar. If the cupcakes were there, would you eat that sugar?

Yes, absolutely. My brain knows what the right foods are. The issue is, how can you satisfy the craving your body is telling you it wants without losing control?

You say something in your body has to satisfy a craving. How is that different from an addiction?

It probably isn't. It just feels different from a societal perspective, right? We push sugar. It's everywhere. It's on TV, the vending machine, at school, every endcap at the grocery store and in Coke and Pepsi or whatever soda is on special. And it's in everything processed, even things you think are healthy or "natural." So, when you're busy and on the go, it's positioned as the easy solution.

How long do you think humans have been eating refined sugar?

Not that long.

Let's say you were a zookeeper and had a chimpanzee. Would you give that chimp a cupcake?

No.

Why not?

It would not make the chimp as healthy as he could be.

It's not what he evolved to eat.

Yep.

So, how are we different from chimpanzees in terms of the importance of eating food we were designed to eat?

Probably not that different.

Do you mind if we talk about insulin for a bit?

Sure.

When we have high blood sugar, we have high insulin. Too much insulin locks our fat in our fat tissues and also gives us that roller coaster blood sugar prompting cravings. So, if I were to say you could lose 50 pounds pretty easily if you lowered your insulin by cutting out sugar, grains and processed food, while being careful with starches like potatoes and rice, how would you feel about that?

Intellectually, I can understand and completely agree. But there's an emotional factor that makes that very hard. It's not that I don't agree, but for whatever reason there's a weird ... I set out to do that, but I'm lazy or cut myself a break or cop out. It's the first week that's so painful or I think I have so much work, so much writing to do. I won't be clearheaded. But in reality, I already don't think I'm as clearheaded as I could be because I know what you say about the insulin is really correct. My mind totally understands it, but I feel reality says I need someone to pack my lunch and cook my meals for me.

A personal chef? OK, let's go back a bit. You said, "for whatever reason" you cop out when you try to go off sugar. What are those reasons?

I'm tired. I've had a stressful day. Maybe I'm annoyed for a variety of reasons, so I feel I'm just going to reward myself. If I wake up and say I'm not going to have sugar in my coffee today, something will happen. I'll think, "You already earned it."

OK, let's say I'm your doctor and I said, "Monica, it turns out you have a peanut allergy. While you don't go into anaphylactic shock, peanuts inflame your body and make you chronically ill. Your body just can't tolerate them." What would you do?

Stop eating peanuts.

So if I said, "Monica, it turns out you have an allergy to sugar and starch. It's making you inflamed and chronically ill." Now what?

It's harder to say I would stop.

If I said, "Monica, you're drinking hard liquor every day. It's making you gain weight, making you tired and wearing out your liver." What would you do?

I would probably go to rehab, AA or some sort of program.

Why is it different with sugar?

It shouldn't be, but it is. I'm not as familiar with a program for a sugar addict.

You feel you would need a program?

I feel I would want to be as clear as possible. There's a degree of support you would get from a program — a way to get support from someone who has been there, done that.

I've read multiple books that basically say the majority of us are sugar addicts. I say yeah that's right, but if there's no action plan that I can actually institute, it's very easy for me to not hold myself accountable for how I eat.

There are groups you can go to for support. Here in our area there's Overeaters Anonymous. There's a whole world of people who are not dieting, but are losing weight through a recovery model. They get the addiction issue. They get the powerlessness over some types of food.

I found this lady who runs a boot camp that's all about eating clean and conquering your sugar and gluten addiction. I think I'm going to try it again. I hope I'll get it to stick. I've known for a while, but I need to get on the horse. I feel I have my mind made up. I don't need a week to start something.

Super. So, are you starting now?

I don't have a good reason not to. I really don't have a good reason. Yes, I think I should.

Wonderful. Please know you can always call me.

For a kick in the butt?

Or just for some pointers. You can do this. Good luck!

Susan W., 62, is a busy and high-spirited teacher in a small school near Silicon Valley. She's 5'1", weighs 174 pounds and wants to lose about 40 pounds. I had been nudging her about my weight loss program for several months, but she was never too keen on hearing about it. After a while, she agreed to a more extended chat.

Tell me a bit about your food and weight problems.

When I was younger, I was as skinny as a rail. My mother complained that I didn't eat enough. When I reached puberty, a balloon popped and from then on I had difficulty and I think a lot of it had to do with the fact that I had a sweet tooth. I also like fast food. I grew up with hamburgers and French fries.

At age 16, I was 18 pounds overweight and went on Weight Watchers, but by college I was back to my old weight. Through college, everything was great until my senior year and truth be told, at that time drugs were big and times were a-changing. But I was not a druggie. I was a food addict. I always felt I had to be in control of myself. Being on drugs would mean losing control, so I went to food instead. It's just that I went to all the wrong foods. I had three skinny roommates who ate like me, but never gained weight. I gained what they didn't, plus more.

After college, I was the heaviest I had ever been. I was 145 and again, I went on Weight Watchers, which kept changing its program, but I lost 25 pounds. I fell in love shortly after and at my wedding, I weighed about 105 and stayed that way for about two years.

But whenever there's a trauma in my life ... I'm intelligent enough to know it was my emotional Achilles heel. I lost my father suddenly at a young age and I had to take care of my mother. I spent six weeks with her after his death and in those six weeks, I gained 20 pounds — the fastest weight gain I'd ever had. I hadn't gone through my own mourning.

I tried to do the things I had to do because my mom wanted to stay in the house and I knew certain things had to be done to have her feel safe in that environment. So I ate. People would bring big meals over and I ate.

After that, I started a master's program, working full time, doing clinical work and I proceeded to gain another 20. Then we moved in 1979 to California and in 1980, I went on something like Weight Watchers. I can't recall the name. A lot of this I think is a gimmick, so you stay a member and pay the fee until you reach your goal. You receive so many points, but you receive extra points a week if you want that piece of cake or that hamburger and French fries. You can do that and still lose weight during the week. Now, what I found is that the weight you lose is much less. It can be a quarter of a pound and everybody's applauding like crazy, and you're sitting there going, "What am I doing this for?"

But I was 167 and got down to 125. I kept that off for a good four years, but then we moved again and I had to find a new job. I found all these things added to when I ate and when I didn't. So I weighed about 170 and wanted to become pregnant. I was 33 years old and the doctors said to me, "All this weight you're carrying at your age is not a good idea."

So I lost 40 pounds again and all the way through my pregnancy I only gained 31 pounds, lost it all after the baby and stayed that way through 1983. And we moved again, so I started gaining again.

More recently in 2008, I joined Weight Watchers again. I got very into it, was exercising three times a week and eating better than I had in years, just in terms of following their program. I dropped a total of 46 pounds and reached 138. But I quickly regained the weight and started Weight Watchers again. I was on it a month and lost ten pounds, but I got busy, stopped and gained it back.

So, you have quite a history of losing weight, but gaining it back.

Yes. It's my eating habits. It goes back up when I'm under stress and when I'm not feeling particularly well. I guess this is stress-related, when I have so much on my plate. And I'm the type of person who makes sure that she pleases everyone.

And you do! So, when you have stress or other pressures, what do you go back to?

Lots of peanut butter, but always reduced fat. I'm a potato and rice liker, lover, actually. And sweets.

What kind of sweets?

Name it! Ice cream is a big one, yogurt is number two, cookies. Anything you have to chew. I'll eat chips, but I'll make sure they're reduced fat, that kind of thing.

When you're stressed, why do you eat these things and not cauliflower?

I'm a big vegetable eater.

So when you're stressed you reach for broccoli?

No. I eat the fun foods.

Why?

They taste better.

Why?

Maybe because of the salt content? I'm a chocoholic.

Do the fun foods make you feel a certain way, say, different from a salad?

The truth is many times I'll be eating it and saying, "Hey Stupid, what are you eating this for?"

But you're getting a different feeling from these foods than when you eat a salad.

There's no question.

Describe it.

I'm satisfying my taste buds? I'm thinking, "Oh, how delicious this is," until I get on the scale the next morning.

I'll tell you what some other people have described and you tell me if it's the same with you. They get a little "escape" feeling, a warm, soothing coating, a buzz.

Yeah, I get that. I agree with that, but it's tainted with, "Look how much you're cheating."

For people like us, would you agree that sugary, starchy foods could act like drugs in our bodies? Maybe that's why we cheat?

Absolutely.

Do you want to change the way you eat, to no longer "cheat" and eat without guilt?

Absolutely. And at this stage of the game, I always worry when I go to the doctor. I'm getting older. I don't want to hear a big surprise. I believe I've been very receptive to colds, infections, GI problems, sleep problems. If I could see that this would help and my head would feel clearer, that would be a big deal to me.

Now, if we cut out all the refined sugar and starches, we will drop our insulin levels and finally lose our weight. Do you believe this? And if so, is this something you could do?

Well yes, and I look at you and I go Ho-ly! But I would say my psyche would definitely have to be prepared to do this. Because I also believe from watching you that it's a lifetime commitment. But, I believe that if I keep doing these kinds of things, I'm going to screw myself up even more.

What do you mean by "my psyche has to be prepared?"

I'm always going to have triggers. What's going to calm me down when I'm working on something? What's that munchie going to be — my trigger foods or if I do your type of plan, a bunch of carrots to chomp on?

What you've told me so far about sweet and starchy food sounds a lot like how alcoholics or drug addicts talk about the substances they depend on.

I have no doubt.

What do people do to overcome an addiction?

They go to Alcoholics Anonymous, they try biofeedback, they go to a shrink, they seek a permanent way to help their addiction in a way they can control or they fool themselves and keep falling off the wagon.

I've gone from one thing to another, had some moments of victory, felt great about myself and then I can't seem to stick on that road.

Not so different from an alcoholic getting sober and then relapsing.

Yes, it's all of it. It's the relapse part that is so difficult.

In all of your weight loss attempts, have you ever fully done away with sugars, starches and grains?

No.

I'm going to suggest then, that though you've cut calories at various times in your life, you've never actually been sober. You've never gone through withdrawal from your white stuff drugs.

True.

Do you think if you stopped the sugars and starches you'd go through withdrawal?

Absolutely.

Are you afraid of withdrawal?

No.

Then why aren't you doing it?

The truth? I haven't bought into it.

Why haven't you bought into it?

I don't know. It's not like I haven't heard what you said, but did I tell you about my earplugs and blindfold? I have a different question. Do some people try it to see if it's for them?

Yes, but as with alcoholics in AA, the ones who tend to be successful are the ones who have support. Would you consider going to OA?

Yes. School's almost out and summertime is the best.

But let's say there wasn't a support group. Why wouldn't you just try it?

That's it! I'm calling you! At the present time, my best support, my husband, we should do it together.

So, have you still not bought into this addiction thing?

At first, I thought it was silly, since I thought we had to eat grains and breads, et cetera, to assist us with our body waste and to maintain a healthy diet. Now, I am being educated to the fact that foods without all those carbs will do the same, especially the veggies. I am truly going to get some support and begin your eating plan and I will be bugging you for more details because I do not know all that you can eat and all you cannot. Slim Susan, here I come! (Laughs.)

Wonderful, call me any time, of course! Thanks, Susan. What an awesome talk we've had!

I thought so, too! Your questions truly made me think about myself, which is not something I do a lot!

◆ Motivation from Jill ◆

When your gremlin rears his ugly head, review this information about what refined sugar and starch really do to your body.

• Refined sugar and carb addiction is real.

• Refined sugars and starches are not empty calories. They are metabolic foreigners that impair our natural hunger, artificially elevate our insulin, create systemic inflammation and trigger fat-generating, disease-building cycles in our body.

• Refined sugar and processed junk foods dull our taste buds, spike our pleasure center brain chemicals just like drugs, and trick us into thinking we can't live without them.

• Sugar and starch addiction is the most pervasive health problem in America today and has led to epidemics of obesity, diabetes, metabolic syndrome, atherosclerosis and heart disease, among other chronic conditions.

• Dieting can result in temporary weight loss, but lifelong normal weight and good health requires recovery from the underlying sugar/starch addiction.

• The body's biochemistry takes only a short time of abstinence and withdrawal to normalize to the point where sugar and junk food lose their former allure and you achieve normal weight for good.

So say BYE-BYE to your sugar gremlin! He's been evicted, ousted, discharged, handed the pink slip and banished! We've wasted enough time, money and angst on him already and there's no room for him in our new lives.

Good luck my new friends! Your recovery is just around the corner and it's well worth the journey. Take it from someone who's been there.

A Handy, if Unconventional
◆ Glossary ◆

USDA Food Pyramid: A marketing tool of the U.S. agricultural industries to increase sales of grains, wheat, rice, corn and soy. Now replaced by the "MyPlate" concept, but based on the same grain-heavy, insulin-spiking guidelines.

Refined sugar: A highly refined, dense carbohydrate that may trigger cycles of compulsion to eat more dense carbs. In the U.S., usually made from genetically modified sugar beets. For millions of years, a substance our ancestors never ate.

Easy: Losing weight through recovery from sugar and carb addiction.

Hard: Losing weight through dieting, caloric restriction or strenuous exercise.

Diet: A miserable thing people used to do to themselves in frustrating attempts to lose weight. And, like wallpapering over a hole on the side of the Titanic, it generally fails to stem the tide. See also *calorie counting.*

Breakfast cereal: Highly profitable concoctions of grain dust, sugar, food colorings and preservatives marketed as "heart healthy," but actually the cause of cardiovascular and other chronic diseases due to blood sugar elevation effects.

Soda: Water + carbon dioxide + high-fructose corn syrup + food coloring = chronic disease.

The Paleo diet: An approach to eating based on evolutionary nutrition that eschews post-agricultural and modern ingredients like refined sugar, grains, chemically extracted seed oils or dairy products. A nice thing to try after or as part of a recovery from sugar addiction.

Low-carb: Depending on whom you ask, anything from the tight restriction of carbohydrates (for example, 20 grams of carbs per day) to diets rich in complex carbohydrates found in vegetables and fruit (for example, 130 grams per day), but without dense carbs like refined sugar, grain and corn.

Obesity: A metabolic condition afflicting perfectly innocent people who are naturally "allergic" or sensitive to sugars and dense carbohydrates. The result is an accumulation of fat tissue that cannot be accessed for energy, leaving the body starving and overweight. Can often be reversed through lowering of overall insulin levels through elimination of sugars and starchy carbs from the diet.

Complex carbohydrates: Leafy greens, vegetables, fruits, tubers (yams, sweet potatoes, potatoes), legumes. Also less nutritious, but more ubiquitous, wheat and other grains, rice and corn.

Healthy whole grains: A contradiction in terms for anyone who is overweight or has sensitivities to carbohydrates or gluten.

Autoimmune disease: A condition often created or exacerbated by ingestion of grains.

Beer and bread: In ancient times, known as slave food. Now thought of as staples. Higher profit margins available for those with labels that look artisanal.

Sugar/starch addiction: The most prevalent disease in America.

Snacks: A form of recreational eating recovering addicts do not engage in.

Dietary fat: Something essential to the human body and not to be feared, particularly in moderate quantities. Healthy fats can be found in butter, olive oil, coconut oil, fish oil, grass-fed meats, lard, avocados, nuts and olives. Unhealthy and potentially dangerous fats can be found in modern contrivances like trans-fats, margarine and seed oils like soybean oil, cottonseed oil, canola oil and corn oil.

Middle age: A time of life when the body becomes especially sensitive to refined sugar and starch.

Insulin: A hormone secreted by the pancreas to help our cells absorb glucose molecules. In high levels, as caused by chronic ingestion of sugars and other dense carbohydrates, it causes fat accumulation, inability to burn fat as fuel and feelings of craving and hunger.

Diabetes, type 2: A sugar/starch poisoning syndrome that causes the body to become insulin resistant and in later stages, to cease production of insulin. A potentially fatal disease that could be solved overnight if the authorities stopped talking about "behavioral changes" and started talking about sugar/starch intolerance, addiction and sugar/starch poisoning.

Cookies: Insulin-spiking and disease-creating sugary, processed thingamajigs sold by Girl Scouts and convenience stores.

Convenience stores: Where addicts go to find their next fix, including alcohol, cigarettes, porn, and processed sugary snacks.

Withdrawal: A process of biochemical repair entailing temporary discomfort necessary to recover from sugar addiction, overweight or obesity.

Depression: A common side effect of eating grains and refined sugars.

Indigestion: A common side effect of eating grains and refined sugars.

Weight gain: A common side effect of eating grains and refined sugars.

Inflammation: What happens to our bodies when we eat refined sugars, grains and industrial seed oils.

Calorie counting: A great way to sabotage a weight-loss plan via ignorance of the profound biochemical effects of sugars and starchy carbs.

Time: What people have more of when not enslaved by cravings for junky food or feelings of guilt.

Money: What people save by not eating processed or packaged food.

Biochemistry, impaired: The reason we get fat.

Willpower, lack of: An antiquated theory about why we get fat.

Shame: Something no overweight person should ever feel.

Addiction, acceptance of: The transformative moment when we people afflicted by overweight can finally take control of our health.

◆ Resources ◆

It would be difficult to list all the resources I consulted as I wrote this book. My research not only included books, articles, research papers and dozens of interviews, but also websites, blogs, videos and podcasts, as well as personal correspondence with experts. If you are interested in learning more about nutrition, addiction and recovery, I recommend you start by looking up work by the following people, beginning with the trove of wisdom found in Jimmy Moore's "Livin' La Vida Low-Carb" podcasts. Please note however, this is only a small sample of the many experts who have contributed to this developing field.

Nutrition researchers, practitioners, writers and thinkers

Nancy Appleton, Ph.D., author of *Suicide by Sugar*

Ancestral Health Society, www.ancestryfoundation.org

Robert Atkins, M.D., author of *Dr. Atkins' New Diet Revolution*

Connie Bennett, author of *Sugar Shock!*

Richard Bernstein, M.D., author of *Dr. Bernstein's Diabetes Solution*

Loren Cordain, Ph.D., author of *The Paleo Diet*

Kathleen DesMaisons, Ph.D., author of *Potatoes, not Prozac*

Michael Eades, M.D. and Mary Dan Eades M.D., authors of *Protein Power*

Stephan Guyenet, Ph.D., Whole Health Source, wholehealthsource.blogspot.com

Zoë Harcombe, author of *The Harcombe Diet*

David Kessler, M.D., author of *The End of Overeating*

Darlene Kvist, licensed nutritionist, host of the Dishing up Nutrition podcast

Robert Lustig, M.D., University of California, San Francisco, whose work is available chiefly in research papers, but his very popular "Sugar: the Bitter Truth" lecture can be seen on YouTube

Larry McCleary, M.D., author of *Feed Your Brain, Lose Your Belly*

Marion Nestle, Ph.D., author of *What to Eat*

Fred Pescatore, M.D., author of *The Hamptons Diet Cookbook* and *Thin for Good*

Michael Pollan, author of *In Defense of Food*

The Weston A. Price Foundation, www.westonaprice.org

Catherine Shanahan, M.D., author of *Food Rules: A Doctor's Guide to Healthy Eating*

Gary Taubes, author of *Why We Get Fat: And What to Do About It,* and *Good Calories, Bad Calories*

Robb Wolf, author of *The Paleo Solution*

Addiction researchers, practitioners, writers and thinkers

Serge Ahmed, Ph.D., University of Bordeaux, France

Nicole Avena, Ph.D., Assistant Professor, University of Florida College of Medicine

Kelly Brownell, Ph.D., Director, Rudd Center for Food Policy and Obesity, Professor of Psychology, Epidemiology and Public Health, Yale University

Elissa Epel, Ph.D., Associate Professor of Psychology, University of California, San Francisco

Food Addicts in Recovery Anonymous, www.foodaddicts.org

Ashley Gearhardt, Rudd Center for Food Policy & Obesity

Mark S. Gold, M.D., University of Florida, College of Medicine and the McKnight Brain Institute

Jeffrey Grimm, Ph.D., Professor of Psychology, Western Washington University

Bart Hoebel, Ph.D., Professor of Psychology, Princeton University

Pam Killeen, author of *Addiction: The Hidden Epidemic*

The Nutrition and Metabolism Society, www.nmsociety.org

Overeaters Anonymous, www.oa.org

Refined Food Addiction Research Foundation, Houston, TX

Jacob Teitelbaum, M.D., author of *Beat Sugar Addiction Now!*

Nora Volkow, M.D., Director of the National Institute on Drug Abuse, National Institutes of Health

• Acknowledgements •

Such a short book, but so many people to thank. Thanks to the many people who encouraged me to put my experience and philosophy into writing. I hope I answered your questions, and then some. I am grateful to the friends who helped me along the way: Susan L., who first enlightened me about food addiction as she carefully weighed her dainty dinner in a Massachusetts cafeteria in December 2008; to Barbara F., who deeply inspired me with her story of recovery; to Erin S., Madeleine R., Jeannie B. and Debbie N. for early comments on my drafts and ongoing encouragement. Profound thanks to Melanie H. for her artistic talent. Thanks to the many people who agreed to share their stories with me. I learned more talking to all of you than from a hundred books combined.

I also wish to thank Antoine B. Douaihy, M.D., University of Pittsburgh, an expert in the field of drug addiction, for reviewing an early version of my book; Christopher D. Gardner, Ph.D., Stanford University, for taking the time to share with me important developments in diet research; Nicole M. Avena, Ph.D., University of Florida, for sharing her sugar addiction research with me; and James Lock, M.D., Ph.D., Stanford University, for talking with me about eating disorders.

And finally, the crew at A Book in the Hand for helping me turn my scruffy manuscript into a polished book, and my husband for his support and keen editorial eye.

About the Author

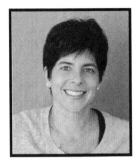

Jill Escher is a businesswoman, autism philanthropist, former lawyer and former sugar addict who lives in the San Francisco Bay Area with her husband and three children. Please follow her blog at www.jillescher.com or reach her at hijillescher@gmail.com.

All proceeds from the sale of this book will be donated to charity.